BUT MY BRAIN
HAD OTHER IDEAS

BUT MY BRAIN
HAD OTHER IDEAS

A Memoir of Recovery
from Brain Injury

by

DEB BRANDON

SHE WRITES PRESS

Published 2017
Printed in the United States of America
Print ISBN: 978-1-63152-246-8
E-ISBN: 978-1-63152-247-5
Library of Congress Control Number: 2017944911

For information, address:
She Writes Press
1563 Solano Ave #546
Berkeley, CA 94707

Cover design © Julie Metz, Ltd./metzdesign.com
Book design by Stacey Aaronson/thebookdoctorisin.com

She Writes Press is a division of SparkPoint Studio, LLC.

Names and identifying characteristics have been changed to protect the privacy of certain individuals. The events depicted are true to the best of my memory.

PRA

But My Brain Had Other Ideas

"Deb Brandon documents her journey with cerebral cavernous angioma, a disease of brain blood vessels, with ferocious honesty. Her tale offers a glimpse into an often confusing and frightening world in which reality can be upended from one day to the next, a world that requires reaching down to the depths of resilience to stay afloat. Brandon's struggles and triumphs will resonate with anyone who suffers from invisible illness and those who love them."

—Connie Lee, PsyD, president and CEO, Angioma Alliance

"*But My Brain Had Other Ideas* is wonderfully written—not only from a literary point of view, but also as a deeply personal and clear explanation of what it feels like to experience the things that Brandon describes."

—Dr. William J. Hawthorne III, PsyD, clinical psychology

"Deb Brandon is analytical, precise, and detail oriented. But her prose reveals 'another side of her brain': authentic, poetic, and romantic. I was singularly captured by Brandon's storytelling. Beyond my perspective as a surgeon and expert on cavernous angiomas, I could not resist hiking along with her in the wilderness, watching her draw from nature the strength to adjust, and readjust. As a professor, I wanted to be with her as she balanced her challenges with the desire to teach and continue to contribute at the highest level. *But My Brain Had Other Ideas* is a lively portrait of the personal toll of brain disease."

—Issam A. Awad, MD, MSc, FACS, director of neurovascular surgery, University of Chicago Medicine and Biological Services

"Told in poetic and exacting language, Deb Brandon's intimate account of life with a damaged brain is equal parts hypnotizing, harrowing, and inspiring."

—Michael Paul Mason, author of
Head Cases: Stories of Brain Injury and Its Aftermath

"Disability does not discriminate; it can be joined in the blink of an eye or in this case a rupture in the brain. *But My Brain Had Other Ideas* is a mind-boggling, roller coaster reality ride of personal trauma, disability, and society's mind-numbing response."
—Lawrence Powell, past director of the Office of Disability Resources, Carnegie Mellon University

"Deb Brandon is more than a remarkable writer and brain injury survivor: she is a voice that needs to be heard by parents, educators, and physicians. Brandon allows readers to experience her most personal and terrifying moments. Brandon's anecdotes, written in fluid prose, emphasize the importance of nonjudgmental support to brain injury victims. I am awed by Brandon's pursuit of a 'new normal.' The human spirit is strong in Deb Brandon. Do not miss this inspiring read by an honest and talented survivor."
—Kelly B. Darmofal, author of *Lost in My Mind: Recovering from Traumatic Brain Injury (TBI)* and *101 Tips for Recovering from Traumatic Brain Injury: Practical Advice for TBI Survivors, Caregivers, and Teachers*

"I know firsthand the challenges you face when you are forsaken by your own body, and Deb Brandon's descriptive prose provides an up-close, personal journey through the diagnosis of cavernous angioma, as well as her ultimate victory in reclaiming her life."
—Julia Fox Garrison, motivational speaker and author of *Don't Leave Me This Way*

"Deb Brandon's memoir, *But My Brain Had Other Ideas*, is a bravely written personal account about her unimaginable struggles with a little understood brain irregularity. Brandon writes honestly about the details surrounding the alarming symptoms, which eventually turned out to be cavernous angiomas, tiny clusters of malformed blood vessels in her brain. Even more horrifying is the fact that many in the medical community initially dismissed her symptoms—which were due to potentially life-threatening brain hemorrhages. Brandon's steadfast determination to not ignore the growing physical complications is what ultimately saved her life."
—Su Meck, author of *I Forgot to Remember: A Memoir of Amnesia*

For Daniel and Sarah

contents

At the turn of the millennium, I was introduced to an illness called cavernous angioma: my infant daughter suffered a major brain hemorrhage leading to her first, horrific and traumatic, emergency brain surgery. Our lives have never been the same. Cavernous angioma isn't an illness that develops gradually, like heart disease or arthritis or diabetes. As with my daughter, it's an in-your-face event—a brain hemorrhage or seizure—that leads to the diagnosis. Once the diagnosis occurs, there is never a safe time, a relaxed time. Sometimes we forget, but a headache, a flu, an odd twitch can bring back the entire history of illness and hospitalizations. The risk of hemorrhage is always there, with no way to predict when it will happen.

Cavernous angiomas are defects existing in the smallest blood vessels in the brain and spinal cord. These lesions are missing essential supporting layers and develop into leaky, mulberry-shaped clusters. They start as pinpoints, invisible to all but the most sensitive imaging, but over time, they grow. If the growth happens slowly, as is typical, it's possible for them to remain silent. It's not unusual to be newly diagnosed with multiple lesions the size of grapes scattered throughout one's brain that have been growing for years.

But then there are hemorrhages, the events a person with a cavernous angioma fears most. Over a span of hours or, at most, a few days, a hemorrhage can cause a pinpoint lesion to balloon, often to the size of a golf ball. Symptoms may start slowly but can become incapacitating—lost sight, paralysis, seizure—or fatal. It's a medical crisis.

A hemorrhage marks a decision point: brain surgery or

leave it alone? Lesions that hemorrhage—bleed—have a very high likelihood of hemorrhaging again and again. The only treatment we have at the time of this writing is invasive brain surgery. For some people, surgery is an option; for others, because of the delicate location of the lesion and possible consequences, it's not. It's hard to fathom, but in the Angioma Alliance community, those who are allowed to have brain surgery are considered lucky.

By my daughter's sixteenth birthday, she was a high school sophomore and had had four brain surgeries. A naive life of reckless abandon is not possible for a person with cavernous angiomas, even for a teenager. The first hemorrhage steals invulnerability and instills caution. We escape in our own ways, because existing naked, steeped in the reality of her sixty brain lesions, would be paralyzing. We live each moment we can in the precious but poignant present.

When I think of the brain, I view it as the structure that defines me most. It's where my thoughts are generated. It carries my memories. It helps me define my goals and purpose. But cavernous angiomas are masters of disruption. From one day to the next, we go from leading our normal lives to facing a future shaped by a bloody brain. Without a doubt, a cavernous angioma hemorrhage is a medical crisis, but for many adults, it also triggers an existential crisis. Who am I now that my brain is unpredictable? Who am I now that I've lost abilities I've always taken for granted? What is my worth? Grief is followed by necessary adjustment to a new normal.

Yet a passionate life is very possible, perhaps even probable. Cavernous angiomas present an unexpected gift: the opportunity to develop a mature understanding and acceptance of what it means to be human and to share this personal insight so that others may benefit.

Angioma Alliance is the patient advocacy and research foundation I started when my daughter was a toddler. My original purpose for the organization was to allow families touched by cavernous angioma to meet online. I didn't want my daughter growing up never knowing another child with the illness. Rare disease can be physically isolating, but the advent of the internet allowed for connection with strangers who became friends because of shared struggles and triumphs. A woman in Ottawa, herself a patient, comforted a wife in Sydney on the loss of her husband. A father in Jakarta reached out for advice on finding a knowledgeable medical consultant. Two families in the same city in Virginia found each other and now spend holidays together. Angioma Alliance created a space that people all over the world have filled with their shared need and mutual support.

By the time I met Deb Brandon, the organization's mission had expanded to include research. As with most of my Angioma Alliance relationships, I initially came to know Deb virtually through our community forum and e-mail, and then on the phone. She reached out to Angioma Alliance to become a research subject and to get answers to her questions about her family's genetics. Without spoiling her story, I can say that there were tests with complicated logistics followed by frustrating results. Even the best scientific methods don't always provide answers. However, Deb's enthusiasm for the work and her support for our search for non-surgical treatments hasn't dulled.

In 2012, my daughter and I took a five-month drive around the country, visiting patient families face-to-face. One of our stops was in Pittsburgh, where we were able to spend the evening with Deb, a friend of hers, and two other families, all of whom were meeting for the first time. It didn't take long for me to learn from Deb about the magical healing powers of dragon boats. I also learned how a math professor, or at least this math professor, compensates after brain injury—very well, thank you.

But My Brain Had Other Ideas serves as a testament to Deb's resilience, to moving beyond simple recovery from brain surgery to transformative redefinition. Her brain may have had other ideas, but Deb's determination illuminates a path for others who face life-changing illness.

—CONNIE LEE, president, Angioma Alliance

prologue

I WAS HALLUCINATING FROM THE ANESTHESIA, BUT I DIDN'T recognize the hallucinations for what they were. I had no frame of reference, nothing to give me direction. There was no light at the end of the tunnel, since there was no end to the tunnel. There was no tunnel.

I remembered being a kid at the beach, tumbling around in the waves, not knowing which way was up, not knowing when I'd be able to take my next breath of air. I felt the same disorientation now.

When I was a kid, I trusted the waves to toss me onto the shore before it was too late, even though their play was a little too rough at times. It was like playing chicken. The fear was delicious, and I went back for more.

There was nothing delicious about this fear.

chapter one

It Was Supposed to Be Two

I WINCED AS THE NURSE-PRACTITIONER, SNIPPING AND tugging at my stitches, caught some hair. She apologized as she worked on another stitch.

I smiled. "No worries—nothing can bring me down now. I get to go home tomorrow."

After two brain surgeries and a week of intensive and much-needed rehab, I was more than ready to be discharged.

As she collected the debris from my stitches, I mentioned that, starting that morning, I'd been hearing an echo whenever I talked. It was an odd sensation.

She glanced sharply at me. "Have you been swallowing a lot?"

I nodded.

"What does it taste like?"

I swallowed. "Salty."

"Do you have a cold? Or allergies?"

I sniffed experimentally, swallowed again, and shook my head.

"Try tilting your head forward. Now back. Is there more to swallow?"

I did have much more fluid going down the back of my throat; I did need to swallow more.

"Try it again."

The same thing happened.

"It's a CSF—cerebral spinal fluid—leak, probably from the site of the second brain surgery," she said. "They usually heal themselves."

Something is very wrong.

A wave of overwhelming fatigue washes over me. I fight to keep my eyes open. *Am I about to have a seizure? I need help. Where is the call button?* I don't see the button. All I see is its cord.

My arm feels impossibly heavy. I stretch out my hand, grasp the cord, and pull on it. It won't budge. I pull harder. It still won't move.

I call out to my roommate and her visiting daughter.

My voice is too small. They are both caught up in the litany of complaints pouring out of my roommate's mouth.

I roll onto my stomach. My head and arm dangle over the side of the bed. The call-button cord is caught on something. I stretch out my arm. I lean. I lean farther, and farther again, another fraction of an inch, and . . . I grab the cord and pull it free.

I press the button, collapse onto the bed, and wait. Nothing happens. I press the call button again. Nothing.

I struggle to think. *I have to get help. I have to get a nurse. I have to get to the nurses' station. I have to get up.*

I roll to a sitting position. I pause to gather the energy for my next move. I launch myself toward the wall. When I reach it, I lean heavily on it. I pause to steady myself. I take a deep breath, press my shoulder against the wall, and slide my way along the wall toward the door, propping myself up with my shoulder.

I rest right in front of the wide gap in the curtains drawn around my roommate's bed, hoping they'll notice me.

But they don't.

Giving up, I move on. I pause when I reach the door. I hear voices coming from the nurses' station.

The hallway is empty.

Grabbing the doorframe, I heave myself across the doorway. I eyeball the distance to the nurses' station.

I slide along the wall, focusing on each step. *Pick the right foot up, move it forward, plant it on the ground. Pick the left foot up, move it forward, plant it on the ground.*

My shoulder runs up against something. I look up—I am a doorframe away from my goal. The nurses have their backs to me. They are still chatting. I try to call, but all that comes out is a soft, halting murmur.

I don't have enough energy to lurch across another open doorway. When I focus to measure the chasm with my eyes, I realize that I'm in luck—the door is closed.

I maneuver past the protruding doorframe, inch by inch, ridge by ridge. When I reach the door, I shuffle across it, no longer able to pick up my feet. I work my way past the frame on the other side. I glance up. Two nurses are sitting six feet away from me, the closest one with his back to me. I can see the other nurse's profile. I breathe a sigh of relief. *She'll see me.*

She doesn't.

I slide along the last stretch of wall, energy almost depleted. I'm barely within arm's reach of the male nurse, but I am invisible.

Leaning heavily against the wall, I slide toward the nurse and tap his shoulder. I whisper, "I don't feel . . ." He whirls around, leaps from his chair, and shoves it under me as I collapse.

It seems awfully bright in the room. My eyes are closed. I try to open them.

I can't.

I sense a lot of people in the room with me. I feel the air move as they move.

I recognize the anguished voice of a nurse I chatted with earlier. "But I don't understand. I was talking to her this morning; she was fine."

I want to reassure her. I want to tell her that I *was* fine when I talked to her. I don't want her to feel guilty; it's not her fault.

But I can't.

I hear a piercing beeping, followed by a tinny voice announcing over and over again something about a code. *Oh, there's some sort of medical emergency going on.*

Why is the light so bright? Am I in surgery?

"She's going into convulsions!"

Who's going into convulsions? I feel a hand on my leg. *Oh, I'm going into convulsions.* I hear the sound of someone moaning. *Is that me? Maybe I'm the medical emergency.*

The light is brighter, though no longer blinding, no longer harsh. It's pure white light, far above me, filling my field of vision.

I want to know it. I want to be one with it. I'm floating toward it, lying horizontally, facing upward.

I'm content. Peace surrounds me, from without and within.

I am.

I am suspended in time. Time is meaningless. I can keep drifting toward the light forever. It feels right.

I continue to float, but . . . the light is no longer drawing me in.

I don't understand. Did I forget something? Is something missing? But . . . I don't . . . I want . . .

My eyes open to a darkened room.

Where is the light? Why is everything so dark? Where are all the people? Even my obnoxious roommate is gone.

Nurses and doctors swarm into the room. Someone says, "You're going to the ICU."

This was not how I imagined my life.

I was an academic, a successful professor of mathematics at a prestigious university. I was multi-lingual, thanks to my international upbringing. I loved to travel, especially to developing countries where I could explore traditional textile work, enriching my own abilities as a weaver. I was the married mother of two young teenagers; we lived a comfortable life in the suburbs. I was young, barely in my forties, and healthy, with a healthy lifestyle. I'd had no car accident, concussion, or stroke. A year ago, no one would have considered me at high-risk for brain injury.

I was not supposed to be here.

I am in bed on my side, with wires and tubes attached to me. One tube protrudes from the small of my back.

Without warning, the universe explodes.

I cannot see. I cannot hear. My entire world has become pain. The pain has no orientation—it has no location, it has no direction, it has no measure. It defies words.

I am pain.

Another explosion, and the pain intensifies. Now there is orientation, location: it is in my head, and it is beyond excruciating.

The level of my CSF has dropped too low, again.

At the ICU, the doctors agreed that I did indeed have a CSF leak, and they were concerned. If the fluid has a way of leaking out, bacteria have a way of getting in.

They needed to test the CSF for bacteria, for meningitis. That meant a lumbar puncture: lying curled on my side in a fetal position to create a gap between two vertebrae in the small of my back, through which the doctor would insert a needle and draw out spinal fluid for testing.

When we were kids, my older brother, Jonathan, got very sick. I watched him lying on his side in bed, curled up, with the doctor and Dad bending over him. Mum satisfied my curiosity by naming the procedure: *lumbar puncture.*

Jonathan was diagnosed with meningitis. Simon and I weren't allowed anywhere near him. I was relieved that I didn't have to kiss him—meningitis wasn't like chicken pox.

The next time I heard of meningitis was when I was in the third grade. During the summer, Galit, a classmate of mine, died. I hadn't seen her since the end of the previous school year, and she wasn't there when classes resumed in the fall. I hadn't noticed her absence until the teacher explained it. My classmates and I stared at each other wide-eyed for a couple of seconds, and then it was time to take attendance—back to business as usual.

As an adult, I was aware that meningitis could be fatal, and I realized that a lumbar puncture was a major procedure. But I retained my childhood perspective on the matter, a curious sort of naiveté—no fear, no worries, nothing. I viewed the whole event completely objectively. It was simply an interesting experience.

I was preoccupied by my disappointment at not being discharged and by my distress over the fact that my kids would see me in a hospital setting; they'd seen me in the hospital far too much over the past few months.

As I curled on my side into the fetal position, I felt as if my body were not my own; everything was happening to someone else, to a stranger.

I knew I wasn't going to die. The lumbar puncture was merely another unnecessary medical test among many. It was a nuisance, an inconvenience, a waste of time and resources.

The test was negative; I was free of infection. I felt like telling the doctors, "I told you so." I wanted to know if I could please go home now.

The doctors did not share my optimism. Since the needle was already in place, they decided to attach a catheter to it—a lumbar drain.

A lumbar drain operates essentially like an IV in reverse: the drain siphons fluid out of the spinal column into a drainage bag. Before it reaches the bag, the fluid flows through a tube, called a buretrol, which measures the volume of liquid passing through it. A spigot controls the rate and amount of drainage.

The surgeons wanted to remove enough CSF to relieve pressure from the site of the leak to increase the probability that it would repair itself. If it didn't work, we were looking at a third brain surgery.

I believed that the doctors were fussing over nothing. There was some sort of disconnect in my mind: on the one hand, I knew that a third surgery wasn't in the cards, and on the other hand, I was sure that the lumbar drain wouldn't work. But I missed the connection between the two—it did not occur to me that if the lumbar drain didn't solve the problem, I would have to undergo another surgery.

Anyway, none of it really mattered. I was more interested in the potential discomfort involved in having a tube sticking out of my back.

Would I have to lie on my side the whole time? Would I be

allowed to switch sides? Would the various tubes and wires get tangled? How often would the nurses change the dressing? Would they constantly obsess about infections?

One inconvenience that I did not anticipate was the balancing act involved.

The CSF's purpose is to act as a shock absorber, cushioning the brain against injury caused by movement. When the level is too low, it cannot perform its function effectively. If the level drops too far, the brain sets off alarms—seizures, brutal headaches.

The doctors wanted to remove enough CSF to promote self-healing, without lowering the level too much. The fact that the body continually replenishes CSF complicated things. Instead of merely removing a certain amount by draining the fluid in a single step, they had to remove fluid at an appropriate rate, which meant that the balancing act would be ongoing for the duration of the healing process.

The plan was to first remove sufficient CSF by draining it at a faster pace than the rate at which it was produced—but not too fast. Once the fluid was at the optimal level, they would adjust the flow rate to match the rate at which my body produced it, thus maintaining the optimal level. Sustaining such a delicate balance requires careful management, and there's more than one way to do it.

After the doctor inserted the lumbar drain, he supervised the initial CSF drainage until he deemed the level optimal. He demonstrated to the ICU nursing staff how far to turn the spigot in order to maintain an appropriate drainage rate. He instructed the nurses on how to monitor the rate of the flow by tracking the volume passing through the buretrol, and suggested checking it periodically in case minor adjustments were needed.

The nurses followed his instructions for several hours, but then the routine changed. Instead of adjusting the flow every so often, the nurses kept turning the spigot on and off. If the level of the fluid was too high, they turned the spigot off, and when a sufficient amount drained into the bag, they started the CSF flowing yet again. Apparently, they were now following another doctor's orders.

Later, when the original doctor made his rounds, he criticized the nurse for using the intermittent-flow method. He patiently explained that there was a greater danger of letting out too much CSF with the intermittent method, for example, if a nurse was delayed.

He adjusted the rate and repeated his earlier orders.

The nurse nodded and proceeded to follow his instructions. Throughout her shift, she wandered in and out to check the flow rate and fiddle with the spigot to make minute adjustments.

The second doctor came into my room several hours later. He questioned the nurse on the drainage procedure she was using. When she described the first doctor's method, the second doctor reprimanded her. He patiently explained that if the CSF is drained continuously, the flow rate must be just right. It was much easier to determine the correct amount than the perfect rate. The nurse was to drain a certain amount at certain intervals.

The nurse merely nodded and followed his instructions, until the second doctor's shift was over.

Neither method was infallible. The CSF level dropped too low several times during each of the doctors' shifts, swamping my world in pain.

I was sufficiently cognizant to realize that I needed painkillers, and that I needed them fast. I was aware of the procedure I needed to follow to procure the medication. I was not too far gone to realize that I needed to take action, not merely theorize on it.

The fact that I was able to breathe and that my heart continued to beat seems miraculous now. The fact that I managed pick up the call-button device, find the button, and then press it is still mind-boggling. I cannot begin to understand how I was capable of speech, let alone of explaining the issue over the intercom.

I croaked, "I have a bad headache. I need pain meds."

A cheery voice answered, "We'll be right with you."

Then it was time to wait. A mere couple of minutes seemed like a lifetime. When the nurse finally arrived, her voice was gentle. "Here you go."

She held out a little paper cup with the painkillers in it: two white pills. Raising my hand to take the cup was no easy task. Every motion added to the pain, making me wince, which intensified the pain further. Trying to minimize additional agony, I worked hard to keep my motions fluid.

Once I held the cup of pills in my hand, I brought it up to my lips and tilted it toward my mouth until the pills tumbled onto my tongue. I handed the little cup back to the nurse, reached for the cup of water that she held out to me, lifted it to my lips, tilted my head back, took a mouthful of water and swallowed it with the pills, handed the water cup back, lowered my hand onto the bed, and let my head sink into the pillow.

By the time I laid my head down, I was completely drained of energy. I held myself as still as possible, all my muscles tense, my eyes tightly shut, my brow furrowed, my breathing shallow, engulfed in pain.

And I waited for the miracle to occur. I waited and waited, an eternity.

A glimmer of a thought entered my mind: *relax.*

I worked to ease the tension in my muscles, but every movement, however slight, increased the pain, causing a sharp intake of breath, which intensified the pain, causing my entire body to tense up again. I had to focus on breathing slowly and evenly. But concentrating, focusing my mind, also exacerbated the pain, tightening my muscles further.

Relax.

I lay with my eyes closed. I carefully eased the tension one muscle at a time, my toes, then feet, then legs, all the way up to my neck, facial muscles, and brow. I tried to relax mentally. I envisioned gentle waves washing through me, one chasing the other, each wave carrying more of the pain along with it, cleansing me of it.

My mind drifted back and forth with the undulating waves, floating, worlds away from my hospital room. Then, slowly, the hospital setting eased into my awareness. I lay in bed feeling the worn, soft cotton sheets between my fingers, seeing the green lights flickering on the monitor, hearing a distant hum from the hallway. It occurred to me that I had left the pain behind somewhere.

During those first couple of days after I'd moved to the ICU, I spent most of the time in bed. I was allowed only a minimal level of mobility; I was not to leave my room.

Getting out of bed was a major undertaking. A nurse had to remove the wires and ensure that the tubes did not become tangled. Next, she had to hang my bag of "brain juice"—the CSF fluid collected from the lumbar drain—on the hook of a portable IV stand.

I left my bed no more than a handful of times per day: to sit in a chair for a change of scenery and to go to the toilet.

The first time I needed to pee, I discovered good news and

bad news. Given that there was no bathroom in sight, I assumed that I would have to use a bedpan. The nurse who came in to assist me claimed that I'd be using a toilet. I was mystified—no bathroom, no bedpan, and I wasn't to leave the room.

She bustled over to the wall-to-wall cabinets on my left and leaned down to open one of the lower ones, and, to my utter disbelief, a toilet swung out as the cabinet door opened. She seemed quite pleased with herself over the arrangement, as though she'd designed it herself. I was dumbfounded.

I wasn't permitted to shower; the dressing on the drain site could not get wet under any circumstances, for fear of infection. I became proficient at administering sponge baths to myself while sitting up in bed.

I had very little privacy; ICU patients had to be visible at all times through a window overlooking the hallway. Nurses and doctors entered the room at will.

At first, I regarded the lumbar drain as nothing more than a nuisance, but within a few hours of its insertion, it grew on me. It made my life quite interesting. It provided entertainment as I watched the battle over my treatment—the doctors' interactions with the nurses, figuring out which technique was being used, guessing the length of the doctors' shifts based on what the nurses were doing. More important, it provided me with much-needed human interaction. I was starving for attention.

I had few visitors. A couple of the staff members from inpatient rehab came by for a quick chat between patients. My then-husband, Bill, brought the kids in for a ten-minute visit on my first day in the ICU and popped in briefly later on his own, and again for a moment the following day.

Nurses stopped by frequently to check on the quantity of CSF that had drained, to change a new bag for the old, to fiddle with the spigot that controlled the flow rate, and to check the dressing. The lumbar drain leaked a couple of times, requiring some messing around with the tube, a change of dressing and bedding.

Doctors came by periodically to supervise the drainage procedure and to evaluate the effectiveness of the treatment. They'd ask about the status of the fluid dripping down my throat. How often was I swallowing? More or less frequently? The same? Was it salty?

Every time they asked, I paused to think, swallow, and respond. I was swallowing at a constant rate, and it was salty—no change.

I enjoyed the doctors' and nurses' company, joking around with them while they conducted their lumbar drain-related business.

I had no interest in the CSF leak itself. To me, it was no longer an issue. Everything was very much about the here and now. The echo I had heard way back when, a couple of days previously, was gone. Because I was a hay-fever sufferer, having fluid in the back of my throat was not worthy of notice. Therefore, there was no tangible evidence of the leak's existence. It was an abstract notion, not real, which meant that I didn't truly believe the lumbar drain was necessary. I was bored with the ongoing discussions about whether the drain was healing the leak. It brought no change, so the endless deliberations were pointless.

The future was as meaningless as the past. It was irrelevant, imaginary. There was only the here and now, and the only here and now was the lumbar drain—learning to live with it, the nurses' and the doctors' amusing rituals evolving and revolving around it, and the social life it afforded me.

"You need a third surgery. Tomorrow."

My world shrank to a tableau. We were suspended, frozen: the neurosurgeon, mid-stride, his mouth still forming the "ow" in "tomorrow"; Abby, my occupational therapist from inpatient rehab, her head mid-turn toward him, her silky blond hair still swinging; and me, facing the neurosurgeon, my eyes wide, my jaw on the verge of dropping.

For a split second, as his words formed into a sentence, every detail was in sharp focus: the outline of his body against the doorway, the creases and shadows on his blue scrubs, every curl on his head, every stray hair, every strand of his well-groomed beard.

Then the lights dimmed, dulling the colors. All sounds were muted; a heavy, suffocating silence filled the room. The monitors were no longer beeping, all footsteps were stilled, and the chatter from the nurses' station ceased.

Suspended, disconnected, I floated motionlessly like an astronaut in a gravity-free space.

All my jokes dried up.

I was lost.

This was not how it was supposed to be. It was supposed to be two surgeries, that's all—not three. Two surgeries to fix the cavernous angiomas, those tangled blood vessels in my brain that had leaked blood, followed by rehab, followed by getting my life back. Two surgeries that I'd planned for, prepared my kids for, built defenses for.

Two, not three.

But my brain had other ideas.

chapter two

I'd Always Been Healthy. I Still Was.
It Was Just That . . .

THE ROOM AROUND ME SPUN FASTER AND FASTER. I took my eyes off the computer screen, put my head down, and focused on the floor. But the world beyond that patch of stained, sand-colored carpet kept spinning. I tried closing my eyes, which only made it worse. I opened them; the dizziness persisted.

I needed help.

I measured the distance to the doorway. I nudged the chair away from the desk, grasped the armrests, and carefully pushed myself to a standing position. I shifted my hold to the edge of my desk, one hand at a time. As the room continued reeling around me, I lurched around the desk, gripping it so I wouldn't fall. Every few steps, I rested briefly, hoping that the dizziness would desist. When I reached the end of the desk, I stretched my arm over to the wall and continued to the door, my fingers digging into the grooves between the cinder blocks. When I reached the door, I grabbed the doorframe and paused to evaluate the next leg of my journey.

I took a deep breath; then, clinging to the wall, I headed down the hall, toward the secretaries' office, cinder block by cinder block. When I reached the corner and paused again to take stock of the situation, I became aware that I wasn't leaning quite as heavily against the wall. I stood motionless, listening to my body, shifting my gaze to different reference points for confirmation: I directed my gaze toward the wall, then to the floor, and finally to the blue sky outside the window down the hallway. The dizziness was definitely diminishing, and, within a couple of minutes, my surroundings stopped moving altogether.

I walked back into my office and sat down at my computer to finish my work.

It hadn't occurred to me to continue to the secretaries' office to alert someone to the episode, the same way it hadn't occurred to me to use the phone to call for help when it first started.

And . . .

I scan the heads of the students bent over their exams in the auditorium-style classroom. I don't see any other arms raised, so I turn to saunter back down toward the podium.

Still scanning for questions, I raise my right foot to take a step, when the room around me starts swaying as I teeter on my left foot; arms flailing, I manage to regain my balance, my right foot joining the left on the floor.

I pause for a split second, letting my eyes sweep across the bent heads around me. I shift my focus to my feet and experiment by taking a small step. I am still a bit wobbly but not enough to deter me from proceeding down the stairs cautiously. I continue one careful step at a time, resting at any sign of unsteadiness. By the time I reach the bottom, my balance is back to normal.

I scan the room again and, seeing a raised hand, I hustle over to field another question.

Then . . .

On my way out of my bedroom, I notice that my left arm is tingling. I rub it with my right hand as I walk towards the stairs. The tingling persists. Mystified, I sit down on the top step to isolate the sensation and puzzle it out.

Bill happens by and gazes up at me. "What's up?"

I rub my arm again. "I'm not sure. My arm's tingling, and it's a bit numb. It's odd, almost like I slept on it, but not quite. Wait . . . it's stopped."

We look at each other. I shrug, and he shakes his head.

Later that day . . .

I briefly experience some tremors. I tell Bill about it, and he suggests that I mention it to Dr. Knupp the next time I see her.

I described the symptoms to my primary care physician (PCP), Dr. Knupp, at my annual check-up, a few months later.

She sent me for a battery of tests, including a brain MRI.

I was reclining in bed, reading, when she called with the MRI report. I reached over to pick up the phone, and when I heard her voice, I settled back into the pillow.

"It looks like it could be something serious."

I sat up. "Oh?"

I caught only bits and pieces of her explanation. Mini-strokes. Cancer. Neurologist.

How dare he be so dismissive without even looking at the report? Who does he think he is? Does he think I'm a moron? No one treats me like this! No one!

The neurologist entered the exam room and, without having read anything about my case, without even glancing at the technician's report from my brain MRI, had the gall to tell me that there was nothing to worry about.

I was incensed. I had just spent two weeks terrified, stewing and worrying, and he'd dismissed it all without giving me and my case the time of day.

He walked in, introduced himself, and asked me about the purpose of my visit.

I handed him the report as I explained, "This is the tech report that goes along with my brain MRI."

He paid no attention to it. He asked who had referred me to him and why I'd undergone a brain MRI.

I told him about the symptoms that had prompted Dr. Knupp to send me for an MRI and that she had referred me to him after she'd received the report.

He nodded. "She's referred patients to me in the past. She's an excellent doctor."

He then conducted a perfunctory neurological exam. He checked my reflexes and scratched the soles of my feet with an open paper clip. Next, he had me close my eyes, stretch out my arm, and bring my index finger in to touch the tip of my nose. Finally, he observed me as I walked heel to toe.

As the examination wore on, I became angrier and angrier. I got the distinct impression that he thought I was wasting his time.

The neurologist seemed to view my stellar performance on

the tests as proof positive that there was nothing wrong with me, and he reiterated his earlier statement that the chances of anything being seriously wrong were minimal. "Technicians often make mistakes," he blithely reassured me.

My temples throbbed. I ground my teeth. I dug my nails into the edge of my seat, my knuckles white. Livid, I opened my mouth to respond, but nothing came out.

I couldn't believe that this doctor had the audacity to announce that there was nothing wrong with me, basing his evaluation on nothing. He hadn't heard a word I said—I had told him that the symptoms had lasted no more than a couple of days. Given that he had no idea what was in the report, I couldn't fathom how he could possibly make the statement about technicians making mistakes.

His voice droned on. "You're a mathematician—you understand the statistics." He repeated his explanation about why it couldn't be anything serious.

I couldn't bear the sound of his voice. I didn't even want to breathe the same air.

From behind the neurologist, Bill gestured with his hand for me to calm down. I focused on his hand, my eyes following it up and down, up and down, trying to keep my temper in check.

I felt an abrupt shift in the atmosphere. The neurologist's tone of voice had changed. "I'll try to bring up the MRI images on the computer."

Had he caught a glimpse of something in the report?

Still furious, as soon as he left, I told Bill, "Let's just go. I can't stand him. I want to leave right now."

Bill, always loath to confront anyone, said, "Hold on. I have a good feeling about this guy. Let's not be hasty; let's see what he has to say."

A few minutes later, the neurologist came back, reading

through the report as he walked toward us. He looked at me. His gaze softened.

"There is some scary stuff in here."

My MRI showed that I had hemorrhages scattered throughout my brain, originating from multiple lesions that were either malignant or cavernous angiomas. The report suggested that they were most probably cavernous angiomas, which agreed with my neurologist's diagnosis, after he studied the images.

I had multiple clusters of malformed blood vessels in my brain, a life-threatening condition with several labels: cavernous angioma, cavernoma, cavernous malformation, cavernous hemangioma, and cerebral cavernous malformation (CCM).

Cavernous angiomas are distant cousins of aneurysms. An aneurysm is a single blood-filled bulge in a blood vessel. Cavernous angiomas consist of clusters of dilated blood vessels, which form multiple blood-filled caverns, reminiscent of raspberries in appearance. As with aneurisms, the walls of these blood vessels are defective and can leak blood.

Cavernous angiomas are found in the brain or spinal cord, where bleeds can cause serious damage. They can present sporadically, or they can be genetic.

I had cavernous angiomas scattered throughout my brain, some of which had bled. The large number of lesions in my brain was an indication that my condition was genetic.

At first, the doctors were concerned that the larger cavernous angioma was in fact an AVM, an arteriovenous malformation.

Like cavernous angiomas, AVMs are clusters of malformed blood vessels, but unlike angiomas, AVMs are fed by arteries. This means that the blood inside an AVM flows at high pressure and is therefore considered as dangerous as its distant relative the aneurysm, which is formed by abnormal ballooning of an artery. Cavernous angiomas, or CCMs, pose less of a risk than AVMs, since the pressure inside them is low.

I was to undergo an angiogram in the hospital's outpatient clinic. They'd inject dye into an artery and monitor the progress of the dyed blood as it flowed through the vascular system in my brain. Whether or not the blood from the artery flowed directly into the cluster of malformed blood vessels would tell us whether I had an AVM or a CCM.

The sounds coming from the thoroughfare outside my curtain reminded me of a more refined version of the noises one would hear in a busy souk in the Middle East. The hissing of tires on the polished floors. *A gurney?* A metallic rattling accompanied by a silvery clinking. *Perhaps an IV stand being wheeled along.* Footsteps, some hurried, others slow, a few purposeful, a couple hesitant, several in high heels, most with rubber soles. Anesthesiologists talking to patients, doctors explaining procedures, and nurses speaking in soothing tones.

I was alone in a cubicle in pre-op, wearing a hospital gown tied in the back, reclining on the bed, waiting to undergo an angiogram. I had brought a book and some knitting to help me pass the time, but I was too unsettled to read or knit.

The quavering voice of an old woman emerged periodically from the cubicle to my right. "Please, dear, you have to keep it in."

Occasionally she became quite agitated, and then I'd hear

the flapping and whirring of a curtain being drawn, and a younger voice would chime in. "Sir, you must keep it in."

I don't want to know what "it" is.

Every so often, the loud guy in the cubicle across from mine drowned out all the other sounds. He had a repertoire of two or three feeble jokes, which he kept repeating and punctuating with his own uproarious guffaws. The responses to his levity ranged from forced laughter to nervous chuckles.

Eventually, the corner of the curtain to my cubicle was lifted and the bald head of a male nurse poked through. "Mrs. Brandon, I need to shave you now."

Shave! Why? They're not supposed to inject the dye directly into my head, are they?

"Or would you prefer a female nurse to take care of it?"

What the . . . Oh. I get it.

To perform an angiogram, a catheter is inserted into an artery through a small incision in the groin. They needed to shave my groin area.

I was startled to hear myself say, "Yes, please."

What is wrong with me? My gynecologist is a man, for crying out loud.

"Perhaps you'd like to use the bathroom first?"

I didn't really need to pee, but when in doubt and there's a bathroom nearby . . . "Yes, please."

I slipped on the rubber-soled socks that came with the hospital gown. They felt like a coating of plastic on my feet, and the sensation intensified as the rubberized soles sucked at the floor.

I tried to hold my gown closed in the back, hoping to ensure some semblance of modesty as I made my way across the busy hallway. I wasn't completely successful, so I scuttled over as quickly as I could, squeaking with every step as the rubber pulled away from the linoleum.

When I was ready to exit the bathroom, I checked that no toilet paper stuck to the gummy soles, held my gown closed in the back, opened the door a crack, and peeked out. When I saw that the coast was clear, I scuttled back over to my cubicle.

Shortly after I lay back down, a female nurse came in to shave me.

I'm not sure what happened next. I have a vague memory of being given something intravenously; it did not put me to sleep but made me fuzzy around the edges. A muscle relaxant, perhaps?

The next thing I remember is lying on a table in surgery, surrounded by medical personnel, all of us focusing on a monitor. The neurosurgeon was pointing at it with a latex-gloved hand, his index finger tracing one of the blood vessels. I was woolly minded, everything a bit of a blur, except for the tip of that finger and the path the dye was taking as it flowed through my brain, a muddy, meandering river branching off into numerous tributaries. My muzziness was tinged with a hint of puzzlement: the flow was in the wrong direction, from the river into the tributaries.

I became mesmerized by the sight of the brown fluid coursing through blood vessels in my brain. Not only could I see it, but I could also feel it: as the dye flowed through my veins, it left a tingling trail of warmth and well-being.

I was disappointed when the show was over and the crowd dispersed. There'd been such a lovely feeling of camaraderie as we'd all watched that monitor.

After the catheter was removed, the male nurse wheeled me on a gurney into the hallway, my recovery room.

Since they had cut into an artery, I was to lie with my leg straight and as still as possible for a couple of hours.

Shortly after the nurse parked my gurney and left me, my bladder acted up. It was almost instantaneous. There was no intermediate slight tingling sensation, no negligible pressure that you can ignore and maybe it'll go away, at least for a while. There was no ignoring this one.

My bladder was insistent; the pressure was increasing. *I need to pee. I can probably wait a couple of hours. I don't think so. But I'm not supposed to move. There must be a way. I'll ask a nurse. No, I can make it.*

Every so often a nurse would stop by, take a peek at the dressing, and ask how I was doing.

The urge to pee escalated to an I-need-to-go-to-the-bathroom-now situation. If this had been an early-morning need while I was luxuriating in bed, I would have been unable to deny it any longer and would have gone to the bathroom right then and there. The next time a nurse checked on me, I told her about my plight.

"I'll get you a bedpan."

A bedpan! Yuck! I have to do it here? In the hallway? No way!

"That's okay. I don't need to go that badly. I can wait."

"Are you sure?"

I nodded vehemently.

But my bladder was relentless. I had to keep reminding myself not to wriggle, not to squeeze my thighs together. My entire being was focused on the muscles between my waist and my knees. I had to fight hard, I couldn't relax, I couldn't allow even one drop to escape, or it would all come gushing out. No use; I couldn't wait even a few minutes, let alone more than an hour. The next time she came by, I asked the nurse for a bedpan, my apologetic smile more of a grimace. When she came back with it, she brought the male nurse with her. As he very carefully lifted my bum up a few inches, she deftly slid the bedpan beneath it and covered it all with a sheet. *Is the sheet doing the trick? Can anyone tell that I have a bedpan under me?*

I had expected the bedpan to be cold and cumbersome; it was not cold, nor was it overly unwieldy. It was flatter, shallower than I had anticipated, to the point that I was concerned that there would be a spill, despite the lip's being rounded inward. *Oh. A splash guard.*

I was apprehensive about putting too much weight on it and tried to lie on it gingerly, but I realized I wouldn't be able to hold out that way. I thought that it might actually be painful having the hard surface digging into me for too long, but as I put more weight on it, I found that the gently contoured edges eliminated that problem. I worried that having my back arched over it would become unbearable after a while, but the flatness of the bedpan minimized that issue.

It wasn't too, too bad. It certainly was not as bad as I had foreseen, though it was so unnatural and . . . actually, it was pretty uncomfortable having a large, hard lump under me while I was supposed to stay as still as possible, and though only slightly, my back was arched, which was definitely not a great position to hold for more than a couple of minutes.

And what if it spills over my thighs? What if it wets the dressing on the incision? How can I make sure it'll go into the bedpan? How does this work? There's no way I can pee like this. I'd never peed lying down, and there was so much going on around me. *And all these people . . . I'm sure they know I'm on a bedpan. I bet all the nurses know. And they're bound to hear it when it comes out.*

I tried to relax, but I just couldn't do it. Whether it was because of the physical discomfort or my prudishness, I don't know. I'd certainly done my share of peeing behind trees. *But that's exactly the point. Behind trees!* I'd never peed out in the open, with doctors striding by, nurses checking on me, patients on gurneys being wheeled past me, some of them staring. And never in such close proximity to strangers that they could hear every nuance of the experience: the rush of the pee gushing out, the splash as it hit the bedpan . . .

The nurse returned. "Any luck?"

I shook my head and blushed.

"Let me give you a bit more privacy." She placed screens around my gurney, patted me on the leg, and disappeared.

I let out a sigh. It wasn't exactly private. The constant activity around me was still very much in evidence. Not only could I hear everything that was going on, but, every so often, something or someone would make contact with my screens, dislodging them slightly from their original position. But it was definitely an improvement.

I tried to envision my muscles loosening. I chanted softly to myself, "Splish, splash, splish, splash."

Just as I felt like I was coming close, my muscles relaxing, the pressure moving toward the urinary tract, a hint of dilation, the male nurse popped his head in. "How are you doing?"

I felt like screaming but managed to control myself and shook my head wordlessly. He retreated and closed the screen behind him. A group of doctors stopped just outside my flimsy enclosure for a discussion. *For crying out loud! Can't you move on a little bit, just out of earshot?* My bladder felt as if it was going to burst. *Just ignore them; they don't even know you're here.*

Again I tried to relax, but just then, the neurosurgeon stopped by to explain the results of the angiogram. "Good news. It looks like it's not an AVM, just a CCM."

This is totally bizarre. I'm having a serious discussion with a doctor while I'm on the toilet. I barely contained my frustration, but with clenched teeth I politely nodded and thanked him. When he finally left, leaving a gap between two of the screens, I took a deep breath, consciously relaxed my muscles one group at a time: my feet, my legs, my buttocks, my stomach. It was working! I could feel a hint of dilation. And . . . I froze.

Another patient was staring at me through the gap between

two screens. I glared at her, willing her to shift her attention elsewhere. But she just wouldn't take her eyes off me.

At that point, my body gave up. My bladder was incapable of keeping it in any longer; the pressure had become unbearable. And the pee came gushing out noisily, in as strong a stream as I'd ever experienced, and through it all I stared that woman straight in the eye.

The good news, that I did not have an AVM, didn't take away from the fact that I had a life-threatening condition: CCMs scattered throughout my brain. I was extremely anxious during my follow-up appointment.

I sat on the exam table, fidgeting. "How will I know if they bleed again? What symptoms should I watch out for?"

The neurosurgeon smiled. "Oh, you'll know, all right."

He then added, "Chances are that you're in the clear. It was probably a one-time deal."

Six months later, I proved him wrong.

chapter three

_____

All Hell Breaks Loose

I NEED TO GET OUT OF HERE. *BUT HOW? WHERE?* MY EYES are pricking with tears. *I can't cry—not in front of everyone!* It is so crowded, so many bright colors, so much motion. *They're too loud; they're too close!* I have to get out. I feel raw, in pain.

My eyes dart around the room. *Where is the door? Why can't I find it? I know it's here somewhere. It's got to be in that direction, or is it that way? Think! Think! Why can't I think? What's happening to me? What's wrong with me?*

The crowd surrounding me is a roiling boiling blurry mass. I can't see past them, they're moving too fast, it's too noisy, I can't focus, I can't single out individual faces, I can't pick out individual voices.

I need to get out. I don't know what to do. I need help. I scour my surroundings trying to slow the world down, trying to make sense of it, trying to find an anchor, something to ground me. I need to find help, but I can't focus sufficiently to seek it out myself. I need help to come to me; I need someone to notice me, to realize that I'm in distress. *But who? Everyone is so busy, no one will notice.* My friends Linda and Cheryl would have noticed, but they're already gone. I would be gone, too, if Dinah hadn't snagged me.

Dinah . . . *Wait! Her voice—I can hear it.* I can distinguish her voice from within the cacophony—my anchor.

Oh, yes, Dinah wanted to thank me for the bracelet, but then someone interrupted us. And as I waited for them to finish talking, the world came crashing down around me, ensnaring me, trapping me deep within a nightmare. I knew that I needed to leave, but something prevented me from doing so. What was it? *Oh, yes, Dinah was holding my hand.* I couldn't let go, it would have been rude, and by the time I realized that rudeness was the least of my worries, I didn't know how to let go.

I feel her hand warm in mine. I hear her voice still talking to . . . whom? The world slows down somewhat, but it is still a blur and I can't make out distinct shapes. I try to turn my head to look at Dinah and whomever she's talking to . . . *I can't move! Why can't I move? What's going on?* But I can move my eyes; they continue to dart around, frantically searching for an escape, for help. I feel Dinah's grasp loosening. *No! No! Don't let go! I'll plummet into the abyss.* I manage to squeeze it imperceptibly, trying to hold on. She squeezes back, and her hold becomes firm again. The tension inside me eases up a touch; I've bought myself some time. *I've got to get help before she lets go.*

I search within my field of vision, but there are no individuals in the blurry chaos around me. I let my eyes sweep across the crowd again and again, seeking a familiar face, hoping.

Decades later, Sandra's face swims into focus and she's looking directly at me! But I cannot speak, I cannot ask for help. I implore her with my eyes, and after a gargantuan effort I manage to mouth, "Help!" I see recognition in her eyes, I see understanding, but then she turns away and disappears into the melee. *Where did she go? Why did she go? I know she understood. I'll cry—I know I will. But I mustn't.*

I don't have much left in me to keep me from tumbling over

the edge. I'm having trouble hanging on to Dinah's hand. It's slipping from my grasp; I'm beginning to have trouble feeling it.

Just as the tears are about to spill over, my friend Cindy's face appears out of the blur. I feel some of the tension leave me. She is moving closer. I sigh. I know that I have the strength to hold on until she reaches me. Right when Dinah releases my hand, Cindy arrives by my side and puts her arm around my shoulder. I'm safe.

I hear her voice from far away. "What's going on?"

I can't answer. The words are too heavy; they can't float up to the surface. All I am capable of is an imperceptible headshake.

She asks, "Do you need to get out of here?"

I manage a subtle nod.

She starts guiding me away from Dinah, toward the exit. *Oh, so there it is. How could I have missed it?* But as she steers me away from Dinah, I become frantic again. *I mustn't leave Dinah, it would be rude, she was talking to me, I need to excuse myself. But I can't talk.* I let Cindy lead me away. There are so many people between us and the door. I balk. *I can't walk past them, they will be too close, they will brush against me, they will talk too loudly. And the colors they are wearing are too bright, blinding, painful.* I pull back. Cindy looks at me askance. I shake my head. I flinch as someone sweeps past me.

She pulls me more firmly toward the door. I make myself as small as I can and try to get closer to Cindy, and, slowly, step by shuffling step, I make my way across the room, flinching every time someone comes too close, averting my eyes when the bright colors assault me too harshly.

Our journey to the door seems unending, and by the time we finally reach it, I feel bruised and battered.

I look down at the plate the waiter has just placed in front of me and smile in anticipation. I've really been enjoying the food in Guatemala.

I place a forkful of scrambled egg in my mouth and almost spit it out. It tastes so bland; in fact, it tastes of . . . nothing. Even water tastes of something. But no—the eggs taste of absolutely nothing. I add some salt. Nothing. I add some more.

I try a piece of melon. It's even worse—no flavor. I focus on the texture; I've never noticed how slimy melons are. I hesitate to try the refried beans. They're not exactly my favorite anyway, and if they're tasteless, too, the pasty texture is going to be really . . . I shudder at the thought.

I say to my neighbor at the table, "My food seems to be tasteless. How's yours?"

She nods, smiling with her mouth full.

I scoop up a tiny bit of refried beans onto the tip of my fork and taste it gingerly. I grab my water and gulp it down, trying to rid myself of the taste of cardboard mush.

To celebrate my return from Guatemala, we order takeout— Thai food. I love Thai food. It's been a while. I can't wait to take my first bite.

First, the dumplings. *Huh. I'll add more soy sauce.*

Next, pad Thai. I always enjoy the combination of noodles, bean sprouts, and peanuts. They form such a wonderful blend of textures and flavors: the al dente noodles soaking up the flavors around them; the crisp bean sprouts, coated with a thin layer of the surrounding seasoning; and, to top it off, the peanut crumbs, adding both crunchiness and a mix of sweet and salty.

Anticipating a pleasurable culinary experience, I lift my fork to my mouth. Cardboard.

I have to find something that will chase away the ever-present nonflavor of cardboard in my mouth. I look through the pantry and spy a bar of chocolate. My eyes light up. *There's no way chocolate can taste like anything other than chocolate.*

I take a bite.

I hastily run my tongue over my teeth, attempting to dissolve the film, but it just spreads it around, leaving a slightly tacky coating of cardboard on my gums, my tongue, my teeth, and the roof of my mouth. I grab a paper towel and spit it out, and get some on my lips.

I search the pantry frantically for something to counter the sensation. I head toward the kitchen, seeking inspiration.

I know! Milk! Chocolate always goes so well with milk. At the very least, it'll wash away the chocolate cardboard.

I raise the glass to my lips and tip it, filling my mouth with . . . liquid cardboard!

The volume on the radio suddenly dips; my hearing becomes muffled. I swallow, but it has no effect, neither causing my ears to pop nor increasing the pressure. I swallow again, harder. Nothing. Once again. Still nothing.

I raise the volume, then raise it some more. *That's more like it. Damn! I missed part of the traffic report. I hope it wasn't anything important.* Luckily, the bridge isn't backed up and the traffic on Washington Boulevard is flowing.

I'm sitting at a traffic light, waiting to cross Penn Avenue, when the radio goes nuts. *Yikes! What the* . . . I grab the volume control and turn it down.

I turn the radio off and continue on my way in to work. When I get there, I just can't settle down. I can't get anything done. I'm too tired. In fact, I'm exhausted. I hadn't slept that well the night before. I decide to cut my day short and go home to take a nap.

On the way home, I start feeling woozy, cotton-woolly, as if I have a bad head cold.

When I turn the key to unlock the front door, I can feel the lock as it clicks into place, but I cannot hear it, though I do hear a muffled bang as the screen door swings shut.

I have a vague sense of foreboding.

Something is wrong. But I can't figure it out. My thoughts keep wandering off and taking the answer with them. I am missing something. I can't quite put my finger on it. Everything feels so detached, disengaged. Bits and pieces of thoughts are floating around, and I can't gather them up and fit them together into anything coherent. I know that a piece of the puzzle is missing, but I have no idea what the puzzle is. I just know there is one.

One of the drifting thoughts I manage to latch onto suggests that I need help to solve the mystery. The next bit that floats by carries the name "Cindy" with it. I make a connection: I decide to phone Cindy. She's my good friend who lives in Colorado, the same friend who rescued me at the big gathering in Guatemala. As soon as I make that decision, my thoughts become a bit more coherent, and I am able to make the phone call and convey some meaning to her, though I have trouble accessing words; I use very simple language, and I am very repetitive.

"Something is going on, but I can't figure it out . . . I don't feel right . . . There's something wrong, but I'm not sure what it is . . . I don't understand . . . I need to figure it out, but I don't understand . . ."

"Deb, what happened? What's going on?"

I tell her haltingly about the hearing issues and the wooziness.

"I'm not sure what you want me to do, Deb. You're not making any sense. Do you need help?"

"I don't know . . . I feel odd . . . I don't understand . . . Something isn't right . . ."

A wave of wooziness strikes hard, as if I have spiked a fever; I feel extremely light-headed and dizzy. I sit down on the closest surface—the coffee table—still holding the phone. "I don't feel too good." My voice is barely audible.

"What? Deb! Deb! Are you okay?"

"I . . . don't . . . I . . . ummm . . ."

I try putting my head between my knees and almost topple over.

I feel weaker and weaker; I have trouble staying upright. Speech is growing more and more difficult; I can't speak above a whisper, and the words are elusive.

"Deb? What's going on? Do you think you're having a seizure?"

I am becoming more confused, and I can't focus on what Cindy is saying.

"Can you hang up and call 911?"

I look at the phone uncomprehendingly.

"What's Bill's number?"

I know that her questions need answers, but I have none. I want to answer her, but the words have gone missing and all coherent thoughts are out of reach.

Cindy's voice is coming from farther and farther away. I can't hear her. I can't hear myself.

Staying upright becomes too hard. I am about to collapse. Gravity and I reach a compromise: I manage to slither down onto the carpet by sliding my bum over the edge of the coffee table, letting my knees fold under me, until I reach the floor. I hold on to the phone throughout—I have no idea what else to do with it. I have a notion that I should do something with it but cannot fathom what that could possibly be.

Next, I find myself crumpled in a heap on the carpet, with the phone propped against my ear. I am no longer holding it.

I lie with my cheek pressed against the carpet. It feels a bit scratchy, like a cheap, nasty synthetic wool blend, and it smells of chemicals and dust. It is covered with a layer of wool pebbles, which are gray, with short brown strands poking out of them. I am fascinated by these brown strands, seeing each one very clearly, very distinctly.

All I can smell is this carpet, all I can feel is this carpet, and all I can see is this carpet. The carpet is my universe, my eternity.

I am completely at peace, in a state of bliss. Perhaps I have attained enlightenment, from a carpet. Who knew?

I feel a disturbance after I lie there for . . . how long? Ten, fifteen minutes? Or perhaps it is half an hour, or more. Something is trying to break into my consciousness, to penetrate the peace.

At first it is a slight disruption, a small ripple on the calm waters, then another ripple and another. Something is trying to make its way across the water, a message. After that thought drifts past me a few times, I realize that something needs to be attended to, possibly by me. But what is that something?

The ripples grow into waves with whitecaps, crashing onto the rocks. Whatever it is, it is urgent. Finally, one part of the message makes its way across. It is followed by other pieces floating on the water. Only a few are relevant. Some are blank; others have meaningless words on them. I decipher the message by snagging the pieces as they float by, spreading them out, and fitting the relevant ones together.

It is like playing charades, or twenty questions.

The message is about Daniel. Daniel is important; I knew that. Why? Then I am filled with a warm sensation: love. Because I love him very much.

The message is about Daniel, whom I love very much. I am lying on the floor, unmoving. That might scare him. I wouldn't want to scare Daniel. Why would I worry about scaring Daniel, and not Sarah? I love her very much as well. Because he would be home soon. Before her. He would be coming home from school, before Sarah. I am still lying on the floor. That is not a good thing. Something has to be done.

I am getting somewhere. I feel proud of myself. But I can't take the time for congratulations. I have to figure it out, whatever "it" is.

I need to do something to avoid scaring Daniel. Daniel would be scared if he found me on the floor, unmoving. I can prevent that. *How? By moving, by getting up. How do I do that?*

I lie there for a while, contemplating the issue. I have to muster up the energy and presence of mind to get up. *I am perfectly comfortable where I am, thank you very much. Wait, what about Daniel? Oh yeah—I need to get up.* But I have been content lying on the carpet. Why would I want to change that? *Oh, right. Daniel. Uh . . . I'm not sure I can get up. There probably is a way; I don't think I usually spend time like this, lying on the carpet. But it really is very pleasant, quite comfortable. Ummm . . . Hold on. I'm not too sure about the comfort part. It feels scratchy on my cheek, it's hard, there's not much give to this surface, and my arm is caught under me at an uncomfortable angle. Actually, come to think of it, lying on the carpet is not comfortable, not at all. In fact, it is definitely uncomfortable. And the phone shouldn't be on the floor.*

I reach for the phone, get up, and place it on its cradle.

"Why did Cindy call the office? PJ came looking for me; I was in the middle of a meeting."

I had no idea that Cindy had tried to contact Bill. *I'm sure I didn't give her the number. She must have looked it up.*

I grin sheepishly. "I kind of collapsed while I was on the phone with her, and I guess she was trying to let you know."

"What do you mean, you 'collapsed'?"

"I . . . just collapsed. I don't think I fainted. I felt weak. But I'm fine now."

"Do you think you need to go to the hospital?"

"I feel fine."

"Oh." He turns away and walks into the kitchen.

That night, I have the worst headache I have ever experienced. I tell Bill that I need to go to the ER.

chapter four

Chaos and More Chaos

I LAY ON THE GURNEY, FADING INTO AND POPPING OUT OF seizures.

I was in the hallway by the nurses' station, just outside the ER, waiting for my turn in the CT scanner.

I was invisible to everyone around me.

I wanted to close my eyes against the flickering fluorescent lights, against the bustling doctors, nurses, and orderlies, against the excited gesticulations, against the confusion. But I was frightened.

I thought that by closing my eyes, I would be relinquishing control of my body to a seizure. I was terrified of the seizures. I was afraid that if I faded into one, I would continue fading, into oblivion.

My eyes closed, and I faded into a seizure.

I lay motionless, having lost muscle tone. But the assault on my senses continued: rubber soles squeaking on the polished linoleum floor, quiet murmuring, excited chatter, agitated voices, monitors beeping, phones ringing, machines humming, the hiss as the doors opened and closed and opened and closed. I felt a puff of air as someone dashed past; I felt a jolt as another bumped into my gurney.

And I popped out.

And then I did it again. I waited, alone, invisible, fading in and popping out.

Finally, it was my turn for a CT scan.

I continued fading in and popping out on my way to Radiology. The fluorescent lights and ceiling tiles rushed past me more quickly than my brain could follow, bringing on continual surges of vertigo. I shut my eyes tight, but I couldn't keep out the sounds. I heard the footsteps beside me squeaking—one-two-one-two—the shush of the wheels on the linoleum, the hiss as doors opened and closed, the clatter as the wheels crossed thresholds.

The reprieves between the seizures became shorter, and the seizures lasted longer.

An abrupt stop, a puff of air. My weight shifted toward my feet. I popped out. And became visible.

The orderly turned toward me. "We're here. Are you all right?"

I nodded.

A nurse and two technicians emerged from a dimly lit room to wheel the gurney inside. They lined it up with a metal table covered with a white blanket, the CT scanner at its head. The technicians positioned themselves behind the table, facing the orderly and the nurse, who were standing on the other side, beside the gurney. Each grabbing a corner of the sheet under me, on the count of three, they lifted me up and onto the table.

"Are you okay?"

I nodded.

Everyone but one of the technicians left the room. He tucked a pillow under my head and covered me with a blanket.

He positioned the table to his satisfaction, took a last look around the room, and left, turning off the overhead light.

And I was alone in the dark, invisible once again.

A huge wave of loneliness swamped me, immediately followed by a wave of fear. *What if I fade while I'm in the scanner? No one would know. I could stay trapped, never popping out. I could die, inside the scanner, alone. I mustn't fade.*

I felt a seizure coming on. I struggled to keep my eyes open. I lost muscle tone. It was as if I were buried alive, isolated from the rest of the world, sealed within my unresponsive body. I had to escape. I had to regain control of my body. I needed to know that there was a world out there and I was a part of it.

And I popped out, my eyes wide open.

A disembodied voice said, "Close your eyes as you go in; once you are in, you can open them."

I gripped the sheet hard as I closed my eyes, afraid that I'd fade for good this time. "You can open your eyes."

And I could indeed open them. My head was in the scanner. Another seizure. My eyes closed and, within seconds, opened with a pop.

I heard a static click. The voice came over the intercom. "Are you all right?"

I swallowed. "Yes, I'm fine."

"Okay, we're ready to get started. Lie still, please. This won't take long."

I pictured Cindy's hand in mine, surrendered to my surroundings, and relaxed.

Cindy lived thousands of miles away, yet the geographical chasm separating us was not as great an obstacle as the ever-widening emotional chasm between Bill and me. Cindy was the one I turned to for support. She gave me virtual hugs when I asked for them, and she held my hand, virtually, whenever I needed it.

It was all I had. It helped, most of the time.

The power inside me switches off abruptly, and I am overrun by fatigue. My head sinks into the pillow, my body melts into the soft comforter, my eyes close. My thoughts drift as I listen to the sounds of the kids downstairs.

I expect sleep to overcome me within seconds, or minutes, but . . . something doesn't feel right. This is no state of pre-sleep. *Oh no! Not again!* I send the signal to open my eyes, to raise my head. But there is no response. *I cannot open my eyes! I cannot move!* I dispatch the signals again and again, but something is blocking them; they cannot break through. Am I comatose? No, my thoughts are clear, and I am very much aware of the world around me.

I fight, continuing to send out those signals, willing them to reach their destination, my muscles. But my brain betrays me and the barriers hold, obstructing their progress. I keep trying, again and again.

I won't give up. I can't give up. I focus on opening my eyes. *If I can only open my eyes, everything will be all right.* I concentrate all my efforts on my eyelids. I aim the signals there and envision propelling them forcefully.

My eyelids are fluttering. Some signals are squirming through cracks in the blockades. But they're too weak after their battle to break the siege, and I cannot open my eyes. I struggle, drawing on my reserves, but I am tiring. I must rest.

I allow my mind to relax, my thoughts to roam. I listen absentmindedly to the sounds around me: the metallic smack as a bat hits a baseball, an engine decelerating and then accelerating, the TV in the family room interrupted by the kids' murmuring voices, Bill's lumbering footsteps, the clock ticking, my breathing, my heart beating.

I feel a mental shift, and somehow I know it is time. I concentrate and transmit the signals, and . . . my eyes pop open. My body is once more my own.

I glance listlessly at the boxes of takeout Thai food; eating has become an unwelcome chore. My appetite, after weeks with no sense of taste, has been essentially nonexistent.

Bill and the kids are eating with great gusto, reaching for dishes, forks clattering, enjoying the food. I don't want to ruin it for them. I've already messed things up enough, every trip to the ER an upheaval, much of my time at home spent in bed, away from them. And even when I am with them physically, all joy squashed out of me by the bloody brain, I often feel incapable of engaging with my surroundings, my kids.

I used to enjoy mealtimes with my family—the conversation, the banter.

I have to make the effort, I tell myself.

I sigh and serve myself some pad Thai. I brace myself and take a bite. And . . . it's good! It's delicious!

I am on the phone, chatting with Cindy. "Nothing new and exciting. Doing anything fun this weekend?"

"Not sure. Might go to a movie. You?"

And . . . I cannot work my vocal cords to form the words. "Ummm . . . uh . . ."

Cindy recognizes the signs. "Deb! Deb!"

"Ummm . . ." I strain to overcome my mental block and manage a whispered, "Tired."

"I'll hang up. You take a nap."

I let the phone fall onto the bed. I lose muscle tone; my eyes close. I cannot move, I cannot see, I cannot communicate. But I am fully aware, and my sense of hearing and sense of touch are intact.

A series of these episodes strike me, one after the other after the other, unrelenting.

Bill rushes me to the ER.

The acronym EEG stands for "electroencephalogram," which is a test that measures and records the electrical activity of the brain. A technician attaches electrodes to the scalp, and wires connect the electrodes to a computer.

EEGs are used to detect abnormal brain activity in order to diagnose medical conditions such as dementia, sleep disorders, and epilepsy.

A twenty-minute EEG yields no evidence of abnormal activity in my brain.

As soon as I arrive home, I head for the bathroom, shed my clothes, and slip into the shower. I shampoo my hair once, rubbing hard, again, and again. I shampoo a second time, then a third. But the glue that the technician used to attach the electrodes sticks firmly to my hair and scalp. Over the next few hours, I pick out the worst of it, one bit at a time.

My hair is gross.

The likelihood that I will undergo more EEGs is fairly high.

It's time for a haircut.

The hairdresser combs out glue crumbs.

"How short do you want it?"

"Boy-short, please."

My breath caught. The wood was gorgeous. It looked as though the grain had two layers: the background a lovely blond color, the foreground ringed with shimmering stripes.

I recognized that blond wood: it was maple, the wood my big floor loom was made of, the loom that I'd purchased from the company Cindy worked for. I was awed by the rings of light, characteristic of tiger maple. I'd never seen anything like them.

I removed the brown wrapping paper completely and exposed the entire piece. It was the cane; the one Cindy had hinted at, that she had made for me.

I sat back and took it all in: the walnut doorknob of a handle, the maple stick, not quite rectangular, and the red-and-black safety strap to place around my wrist when I used the cane.

I brushed my fingers against the wood with a feather-light touch, then ran my hand down it, stroking it. In the warmth of the wood, I felt Cindy's warmth lingering. I could feel the care that went into it, into all the details, sanding it, rounding the edges, fitting the knob on top of the stick, trapping the strap between them, adjusting the rubber tip, and rubbing the oil finish on it.

I pushed myself to a standing position, placed the strap around my wrist, wrapped my hand over the knob, and leaned on it. It was a perfect fit. The knob felt right in my palm. I took a few steps with it. Then I leaned on the wall and straightened my arm to push the knob away from me and looked the cane up and down to admire it. It was exquisite.

The world swam back into focus. The kids were on their way out the front door. Bill seemed to be focused on the cane, like I was, except he had an odd look on his face. Was he unhappy about something? Uncomfortable? I shrugged it off, not thinking much of it at the time; perhaps I'd just imagined it.

Once more, seizures—abrupt, no fading involved, split seconds apart.

Cindy, who was visiting for the weekend, carried me to the car, and Bill drove me to the ER while Cindy stayed with the kids.

The neurology resident questioned me at length about the seizures. He then put me through my paces, testing my cognitive function. He checked my reflexes and observed my reaction to sensory input. He also studied my gait, looked for muscle weakness, and listened for problems with speech.

After administering a twenty-minute EEG, the resident left my bedside with a promise that the on-call neurologist would stop by. He seemed convinced that she would prescribe anti-seizure meds.

I was thrilled. During all my previous doctors' appointments and hospital visits, I had been subjected to one test after another that had led nowhere. None of my medical exams had resulted in anything close to a solution, a way out of this nightmare. Now, finally, it looked like there was an answer, a chance that I'd be able to move on, to improve my quality of life.

After waiting in the ER for a couple of hours, I was told that the on-call neurologist wouldn't make it in until the following day.

I was admitted to the hospital.

Cindy visited me the next morning.

She took in the room, picked the chair closest to the door, and moved it right beside me at the head of the bed. Then she sat down, stretched out, and put her feet up on the bed. She was parked, there to stay.

I was delighted yet puzzled. Did people in this country do that? Or was it just Cindy?

In all my times in the hospital since the brain hemorrhages, Bill had been my only visitor. During every hospital stay, he stopped by daily for a brief visit, never more than half an hour. He always sat on the edge of the chair, fidgeting, making very little eye contact, distracted, frequently glancing toward the door.

Later in the morning, Bill stopped by. He looked more uncomfortable than usual.

He perched on the edge of his chair and turned to Cindy. "I didn't realize you were coming here. I was going to suggest that we come over for a quick visit a bit later on, but you had disappeared."

She shrugged. "You seemed so busy at home, I figured I'd come over to hang out with Deb. When I left, you weren't around. I think you were in the shower."

Bill made small talk for a few minutes and then stood up. "I need to get back. The kids . . ."

He turned to Cindy. "If you want, you can follow me back home."

"Thanks, that's okay—I'm pretty good at finding my way around. I had no trouble finding my way here. I'll stay with Deb."

Bill paused, fidgeted some more, and then left.

Cindy came with me when I went for yet another EEG, and she walked alongside my gurney when I was wheeled in for an MRI. No one had ever done that for me. I didn't realize until then just how lonely and scared I had been.

Later in the day, when the on-call neurologist came in the door with her two-intern entourage, I greeted her with a smile.

After she introduced herself, she said, "I gather you're here for seizures?"

I switched gears and, no longer smiling, nodded. "I had a whole bunch yesterday afternoon, which is why my husband brought me in to the ER."

"Are you still having them?"

"Yes, but at a much lower frequency. In fact, I've had only a couple since I woke up."

Cindy leaned forward slightly. "Yesterday she was having one after the other, with only a few seconds in between most of them."

The neurologist turned toward Cindy and looked her up and down. "And you are . . . ?"

The plastic upholstery on Cindy's chair squeaked as she settled back into it. "I'm a friend."

The neurologist turned back to me, as if dismissing Cindy. "The EEG is not showing anything. Have you had any other symptoms?"

"Well, since the trouble with the angiomas started, I've developed various symptoms. Among other things, my balance is bad, I get dizzy sometimes, I get tired very easily, and I've been getting some terrible headaches. Oh, yes, I've also had neuropathy." I paused and frowned. "I think that's it."

"Thank you. It was nice meeting you." And she walked out. Her two interns followed her, smiling and nodding.

Cindy and I looked at each other. I shrugged, and we continued our conversation where we had left off.

An hour or so later, the neurologist came back, interns in tow. Cindy was still reclining in the chair, her feet on the bed. The neurologist looked at her, frowned, brought over a chair that had been standing across the room, set it against the wall by the door, and sat down. Her interns stood, flanking her.

"I just looked at your chart. You do indeed have cavernous angiomas, and two of them have bled."

I was dumbfounded. Not only had she not bothered to look at my file before she had come in the first time, but she hadn't bothered to listen to her intern's report. I had given the intern all that information earlier that morning.

She paused until I nodded, and then continued. "Are you stressed out about anything?"

My jaw dropped. "Well, yeah! I'd say that having these hemorrhages in my brain have brought some stress into my life."

"Well, you shouldn't stress over it. Your EEGs have shown no abnormal activity. Can you tell me more about these episodes?"

I could feel one coming on; fighting to keep my eyes open was a losing battle. Surrendering, I leaned back and rested my head on the pillow. I spoke softly. "Actually, I think that I'm about to have one."

Within seconds, my eyes closed and I lost muscle tone. As I lay there, fully aware, there was silence in the room, the only sounds drifting in from the hallway.

When I popped out of it less than a minute later, she continued. "We can probably rule out epileptogenic seizures. The seizures you are having are most probably psychogenic, which are often due to stress."

This sounded promising. I had no idea what psychogenic seizures were, but if they were caused by stress that probably meant that they were no big deal. "What are psychogenic seizures? How can they be prevented?"

She looked at Cindy and then turned back to me. "Basically, they are not true seizures. There is no treatment, other than going to see a therapist." I stared at her. "I understand that you are under a lot of stress, that you are worried about the cavernous angiomas. However, there is no reason to worry. They are perfectly harmless."

I couldn't believe my ears. It took me a minute to gather my wits about me. "If they are so harmless, how do you explain the fact that they have affected my balance?"

"You have trouble with your balance?"

Obviously, she had only briefly skimmed my file.

"Yes, I have been going to physical therapy for it. I have trouble only when I'm standing still. Oh, and I can't walk heel to toe without losing my balance. According to my neurologist, I have stationary, um, aphasia."

I was uncertain about the word; I knew that it was either "aphasia" or "ataxia."

"You have aphasia?" She turned to make eye contact with one of her interns, who smiled in response.

I nodded. Since no one corrected me, I assumed that I must have used the correct word. I later found out that "ataxia" was the correct word; "aphasia" refers to difficulties speaking.

"Let me see you walk heel to toe."

I got out of bed and looked around as I leaned against the bed.

"Just walk toward me."

There wasn't much room; I'd have to navigate between the bed and a table. I mentally braced myself. As soon as I placed one foot in front of the other and let go of the bed, my arms started flailing, as usual, and by the time I was about to take my second step I was all over the place. I somehow managed to stay upright for a brief second. About to give up, I glanced toward the bed.

"No, no—keep going."

No other neurologist had ever told me to keep going after two steps; by then it was so obvious that I had a serious problem, there was no need to demonstrate further.

I tried to lift up my foot to take one more step. I could feel that I was about to fall and lunged for the bed. Once stable, I raised my head to look at her. She was staring right at me, frowning. *She looks . . . disappointed? Did she* want *me to fall?* When I made eye contact with her, she put her hands together, the tips of her fingers touching.

"You don't have balance problems."

Once again, my jaw dropped. Out of the corner of my eye, I saw Cindy straighten up, her feet on the floor.

"You don't have balance issues, because you were compensating with your arms."

One of the interns beside her smiled and mimicked my arms flailing. I felt my mouth open and close, but no words came out.

"You clearly have issues. You should see a therapist."

She got up and left the room. Her two interns followed, nodding like bobbleheads and smirking.

Had the stress unhinged me to the point where I was feigning seizures? No! I couldn't be losing my mind. The angiomas were real; the bleeds were real.

But I started doubting myself. *Am I exaggerating my symptoms? Is some of this psychosomatic? Am I an attention seeker?* I knew that it wasn't all in my head, but maybe some of it was. If I tried harder, perhaps I could keep my eyes open; perhaps I would not lose my balance so easily.

According to my regular neurologist, a negative twenty-minute EEG like the one I had in the ER proved nothing.

Had the EEG revealed that I exhibited abnormal brain activity, doctors would have considered it proof positive that my episodes were indeed epileptogenic seizures. But twenty-minute EEGs often yield false negatives.

My neurologist quoted several examples of patients who suffered from severe epilepsy that twenty-minute EEGs did not detect. He explained that the results of an EEG are highly dependent on the placement of the electrodes.

He suggested we try a twenty-four-hour, outpatient EEG. This longer time period would increase the probability of capturing abnormal brain activity.

⌒

"Why are you measuring my head? How do you decide where to place the electrodes? Is this it? This is the EEG machine?"

The EEG technician used a tape measure. Every so often, she drew marks to denote where she planned to position the electrodes.

To my surprise, the location of the suspected source of the trouble had no bearing on their placement; rather, it was determined by calculations based on the patient's head measurements.

She handed me a black box, the size of a high school science textbook, with a carrying strap and a thick bundle of colored wires protruding from one side. I was to place the strap around my neck and keep the box hanging against my chest for the next twenty-four hours.

"Do the different-colored wires have any special significance? What kind of glue do you use for the electrodes? Will it be easy to wash out of my hair when this is over?"

She mumbled incoherently. Perhaps she didn't know, perhaps she was growing weary of my questions, or perhaps, completely focused on fashioning my techno-dreadlocks, she wasn't paying attention to me.

I knew that I was about to be vindicated. I was going to prove that awful on-call neurologist wrong. When she had squashed me so thoroughly, she'd filled me with complete and utter hopelessness. Now, I felt so alive. I felt like me. I hadn't felt this way for far too long.

I left the technician's office smiling, my head held high. I walked with the black box hanging in front of my chest, the bundle of colorful wires leading from the box up to my neck, where they disappeared into a swath of gauze bandages that covered my head, like a mummy's.

The technical report noted a single, brief spell of abnormal brain activity, which, according to my neurologist, was within the norm; the test, in his professional opinion, was inconclusive. I did not feel fully vindicated.

But "inconclusive" didn't matter—my neurologist prescribed anti-seizure meds, because he took me seriously.

After starting medication, I experienced no more episodes until after the first surgery—a fair indication that they had been epileptogenic.

But I couldn't get rid of the self-doubt. Was I being melodramatic? Was I an attention seeker?

chapter five

Heading into May 2007:
This Is No Kind of Life

I SPEAK SOFTLY INTO THE PHONE. "HI."

Cindy sounds concerned. "Are you okay? You don't sound too good."

"It's just a touch of asthma. I've been this way off and on most of the day. I'm also really tired."

Following Cindy's suggestion, I use my inhaler again. Nothing. My asthma has never felt quite this way before. I'm not wheezing, and I'm not really fighting for every breath. It feels as if my lungs and the muscles in my chest and abdomen don't quite know how to function. Each breath is hesitant and shallow. Speaking is difficult; I can't produce enough air. My voice is soft, and I cannot utter more than one word at a time; I have to pause between words to take a few breaths.

"I . . . don't . . . know . . . what's . . . going . . . on."

"You need to get Bill. Can you do that? I'll hang up."

My speech is halting, but my thoughts, though sluggish, hold no pauses. *What to do I'm here he's downstairs I can't yell use the inhaler again.* I roll over slowly toward the nightstand. My body feels so heavy. I stretch out my arm and reach toward the inhaler. It's a couple of inches beyond my fingertips. I retract my arm and use it to brace myself as I shift a few inches closer. Once settled, I pause to rest for a long moment, then roll over again and reach. As soon as my fingers have the inhaler in their grasp, I bring it over to my mouth. I focus hard, trying to suck the medicine into my lungs, but all I can manage is a shallow breath. *So this is what really bad asthma is like.*

I'm so tired.

I wait for an eternity, but the inhaler isn't helping. I try again. It doesn't even take the edge off. That's never happened before; there's always been some improvement.

Thinking is difficult. But I have to figure this out. I need air. *I don't understand so hard to breathe gotta do something need Bill maybe can get Daniel or Sarah they won't hear me what to do.*

And then it registers. The brain stem, among other functions, is responsible for balance, swallowing, and breathing. *Need Bill can't die like this need ER need Bill how to get Bill phone use cell to call him doesn't always pick up maybe his cell off try house phone.*

I roll over again to fetch my cell phone from my nightstand. I press the speed dial for the house phone. I press SEND before I press VIEW. *Damn try again VIEW SEND ringing.* It rings and rings and rings. He isn't picking up. I move the phone away from my ear, peer at the keypad as I use my index finger to press the keys, and then raise it back to my ear. I can hear him lumbering around downstairs while the phone keeps ringing. My limbs are growing heavier. I know that I don't have another attempt in me. *If he doesn't get to the phone in time . . .*

"Hello."

I whisper, "I . . . can't . . . breathe . . . brain stem . . . help."

He doesn't answer. A split second later, the silence is broken by the sound of him thundering upstairs. I haven't heard him move so fast since before his hip surgery last year.

He pops his head in the door. "I'll tell the kids I'm taking you to the ER."

At the hospital, they give me oxygen and keep me overnight. By morning, my breathing is back to normal.

It's almost lunchtime when the attending neurologist stops by. He is totally unconcerned about my respiratory problems, convinced that the cavernous angiomas are irrelevant in this matter. He explains to me that, in fact, angiomas are fairly harmless. Then he leaves. He spends less than five minutes in my room.

A few minutes after he makes his exit, a neurology resident comes in to summarize their findings.

Having recovered from the attending neurologist's whirlwind visit, I am ready to ask questions. "Could the bleeds in the brain stem have caused the breathing difficulties?"

The resident vehemently shakes his head no. "The brain stem can act only as an on-off switch when it comes to breathing and swallowing."

He explains that it wouldn't just cause difficulties; it would make me unable to breathe, just like that, with no warning.

I'm relieved that I probably suffered merely a severe asthma episode.

Two years after the brain surgeries, I joined the Angioma Alliance, an organization that provides support for cavernous angioma patients and is involved in related medical studies. I was participating in a DNA study, and a nurse was interviewing me as part of that.

"Wait, are you saying that you can have trouble breathing when the brain stem is involved?"

The nurse answered, "Well, yes. You can also have trouble swallowing."

"No. What I mean is, I was under the impression that you suddenly stop breathing, with no warning. It's all or nothing."

"That is a possibility, but that's not necessarily the case. We see a lot of angioma patients with respiratory problems due to angiomas in the brain stem."

She told me about a patient who'd had severe respiratory problems from a pinprick-size angioma in her brain stem. Since it was so tiny and had never bled, the doctors assumed it could not possibly be associated with her respiratory problems and for years misdiagnosed her symptoms as asthmatic.

"I ordered you a walker."

All the sounds from without became muffled, amplifying the sounds from within: my heartbeat, my breathing, the blood rushing through my veins.

I heard Cindy's voice as if from afar. "Are you there?"

And I exploded.

I was so furious, I could barely speak. I sputtered, "How dare you? What do you think you're doing?"

Here I was, practically beaten to the ground, and she was trying to rub my nose in it. Did she really think I needed a constant reminder of my plight? Reminders were thrust in my face wherever I went, every minute of every waking hour. A walker would be a symbol of all that was wrong in my life. Did she really feel the need to add to my misery?

Then the balloon deflated, and my anger morphed into grief.

I'd been trying so hard to stay away from the edge, to prevent a fall into the abyss. My life had been reduced to mere survival. I'd resorted to living day by day, hour by hour, minute by minute. I could not handle more than the moment. I wanted to stay blind to the big picture. Denial had been serving me well; it was the only thing keeping me sane.

When my keening died down, I heard Cindy.

She was livid. It was time for me to face the facts. If I wanted any semblance of independence, I had to be more realistic. A walker was a tool, nothing else. A tool that would let me be more self-sufficient. If it was a symbol of anything, it was a symbol of independence.

Bill, like I had been, was angry when I told him about the walker. "Cindy should not have acted without consulting you. That's completely inappropriate. It's not her place."

But as he continued ranting, it became evident that the real reason for his anger was completely different from mine.

"Walkers are associated with old people in bad shape. You'll be stigmatized. The cane was one thing, but if people see you with a walker, they'll think you're handicapped."

Throughout my relationship with Bill, I occasionally had trouble understanding his behavior. When totally mystified, I shrugged it off, attributing it to the social ineptness so common among scientists, or to the differences in our backgrounds and my lack of fluency in American culture. However, since the brain hemorrhages, the frequency of inexplicable actions and reactions had increased dramatically, and I had been having more and more trouble shrugging them off.

Bill's way of handling anything out of the ordinary was to talk about it incessantly. I often overheard him talking at various people about my health, in person or on the phone: his family, his friends, our colleagues, neighbors, parents of Daniel's and Sarah's friends, casual acquaintances. He'd tell them about my latest symptoms, my doctors' appointments, my various meds and hospitalizations. He elaborated on his opinions about what was going on, how I was feeling, and what the doctors were doing. Everyone I encountered invariably knew about my situation. Wherever I turned, I got the sincerely concerned look: eyes wide, they'd lean in, almost invading my personal space, and ask, "How *are* you?"

Even at home, Bill constantly wanted to talk at me about my symptoms, doctor's appointments, and the latest developments.

Whenever I came downstairs, a barrage of words greeted me. "I don't think that you are always aware when you have seizures. I'm pretty sure that at least a couple of times you were out of it. I think we need to talk to Dr. Silverman some more about it. We also need to tell him that you probably aren't aware every time you have a seizure. There were at least a couple of times when I bet you blacked out. We should definitely mention it to Dr. Silverman."

I didn't want to talk about the bloody brain wherever I went. I didn't want to be reminded of it constantly. I didn't want to think about it all the time.

At first, I stayed away from campus as much as possible to avoid my colleagues. Next, I hid inside the house to avoid the neighbors. Then I restricted myself to my room to avoid Bill.

The walker was a deep shade of burgundy. I named her Annabelle.

I didn't use Annabelle much on a daily basis. As Bill pointed out, she was too cumbersome for use inside the house, and even though she folded almost flat, he had trouble fitting her into the car, so we took her along only when it was absolutely necessary.

As Cindy predicted, Annabelle did afford me some of the independence I craved. With the walker, I became able to travel freely, like I used to. Wherever she could go, I could go. I wielded her constantly during trips. I took her with me when I flew to Colorado to visit Cindy, and when I traveled to Boston for a meeting.

She was invaluable.

Toward the end of May 2007, a couple of months after my first trip to the ER, my ER visits ended, but debilitating symptoms continued to plague me.

Now that the seizures were under control, fatigue became my nemesis. I needed at least two naps a day, usually three. During my waking hours, I was groggy much of the time. Fully lucid for no more than three hours a day, I was not capable of much. Handling a single load of laundry exhausted me. Attending one of Sarah's softball games wiped me out. After a trip to the doctor's office, I was finished for the day.

I was not allowed to drive because of the seizures, and I was limited in other activities by my problems with balance and vertigo. I couldn't teach, I couldn't weave, I couldn't wash dishes, I couldn't be a mother. All I was good for were short bursts of activity that hardly seemed worth the effort.

I lay in bed, transitioning out of sleep, my mind wandering.

If I wanted to kill myself, how would I do it? Anything that involves blood, gore, and guts is out. I'd have to do it with some sort of an overdose.

I glanced over to the nightstand, where my meds were, and

started taking a mental inventory. *I wonder if the blood pressure meds would do it. Probably not. What about the anti-seizure meds? It would probably be safer to go with the pain meds . . .*

No.

I was sure I couldn't take my own life. I did not have it in me; I was merely speculating. But my thoughts had strayed a little bit too far. My internal alarms went off, shaking me out of my lethargy.

I recognized that my world had been growing smaller and smaller. I was barely existing.

I could not continue this way. I wanted a life, not a miserable existence. There had to be a solution out there somewhere.

chapter six

June 2007:
No More Waiting

THE NEUROSURGEONS IN PITTSBURGH TOLD ME THAT the risks of surgery outweighed the gains. They would consider surgery only if I suffered two acute bleeds. The little ones didn't count.

We were waiting for the next big one.

After my life turned upside down, while I was still in shock, I was quite willing to place my fate in my doctors' hands. I trusted that they knew best.

Once I was over the initial daze, I didn't want to learn about cavernous angiomas. If I took the time to research them, I would be admitting their existence. I would be accepting the possibility that they were here to stay. But if I ignored them, if I didn't acknowledge them, perhaps they'd go away.

Despite my aversion to learning about the angiomas, some details did sink in.

I had one big one in my right parietal lobe and one smaller one in my brain stem.

They were clusters of malformed blood vessels.

Unlike with aneurisms, the blood flow through them was at low pressure.

Mine had bled.

They had caused balance loss, vertigo, dizziness, seizures, horrendous headaches, hearing problems, loss of sense of taste, confusion, memory loss, and debilitating fatigue.

In my case, the condition was probably genetic, and if that was indeed the case, there was a 50 percent chance that my kids had inherited the illness.

As time wore on and the quality of my life deteriorated to a point where suicide was more than a passing thought, I started questioning the doctors' assessment of my situation.

It was time to educate myself.

Cavernous angiomas are not visible on angiograms. CT scans cannot detect them consistently. Until the advent of MRIs, in the 1980s, the only way to identify cavernous angiomas was during autopsy. Until the early 1990s, when MRIs became readily available, many doctors remained ignorant about them. In addition, since extensive research on cavernous angiomas is relatively recent, many doctors today are yet unfamiliar with the condition, and that leads all too often to misdiagnoses or ineffective treatments.

One neurosurgeon believed that my brain stem angioma was inoperable. His recommendation was that if I had another acute bleed, I should be treated with a gamma knife, a form of radiation-based therapy.

Using a gamma knife on cavernous angiomas is controversial at best. In fact, several highly regarded medical facilities caution against it. There are no guarantees that treatment with the gamma knife will prevent future hemorrhaging, and if the procedure is unsuccessful, the angioma may then have to be removed surgically. Unfortunately, removing an angioma that has been treated with the gamma knife can be more challenging than removing an untreated one; hence, the risk of neurological damage increases.

The chances of a hemorrhage also increase with time, rising on average at a rate of 0.25 percent per angioma per year. I had more than eight angiomas. In addition, the rate is higher during the first two years after a bleed.

Sitting and waiting in itself posed a significant risk.

I researched cavernous angiomas online and read all the books I could find, including medical books directed at medical professionals. The more I learned and the more questions I asked, the less I trusted the doctors. It did not take long for me to feel better informed about the subject than they were.

Until I read *Dipped into Oblivion*, by Sacha Bonsor, surgery was an abstract notion, not a potential reality. The thought was too terrifying, and my mind just wouldn't go there.

A significant portion of the book focuses on the author's path to surgery. Like I did, she had an angioma in her brain stem. Neurosurgeons also told her to wait and see. Like I did, she searched for alternative answers.

Her book was an affirmation that I was not being melodramatic. It validated my questioning of the recommended course of treatment, or lack thereof. It confirmed my belief that other viable solutions were out there, and that surgery could very well be a feasible option.

Her book brought me relief and lent me the strength and resolve I needed to become proactive. It brought control back into my life.

My research, which until that point had had little direction, now concentrated on Dr. Spetzler, who performed Bonsor's surgery.

He had performed hundreds of successful brain stem surgeries. In addition, his expertise lay in removing cavernous angiomas. His success rate was over 90 percent, compared with the nationwide success rate, which was approximately 85 percent.

I wanted a health assessment by someone who was respected by the neuro-community, and I wanted a recommendation for treatment from someone I could trust, a true expert.

I wanted Dr. Spetzler's opinion.

If he advocated surgery, I wanted him to perform it. No one else would do. Unless . . . unless I disliked him.

Bill collected all the relevant documents: the numerous CT scans and MRIs, the EEGs, the various reports from my hospitals stays, and the case history that my neurologist produced. Bill also wrote a list of all my symptoms and a chronology of everything that had occurred from the first symptoms to the present.

We put it all in a large envelope and sent it off to Dr. Spetzler.

Did Bill hand it to me? Did I collect the mail?

I thought I remembered. Now I'm not sure. But as I write, I do recall quite vividly what came next.

I am sitting at my computer table, staring at the envelope, reading and rereading the logo, BARROW NEUROLOGICAL INSTITUTE. I swivel on my stool so that I am facing Bill. He is standing in the doorway.

I look at him for assurance. He nods imperceptibly. My eyes return to the envelope. With shaking hands, I run a finger beneath the flap, tearing the envelope open. I look back up at Bill. He nods again. I pull out a letter and unfold it.

My hands are shaking so hard that I can't read it. I rest it on my lap and breathe in. After I let the air out, I square my shoulders, pick up the letter, and read. I swallow, then reread it.

I raise my head. "He recommends surgery. On both the big one and the brain stem one."

We stare at each other for a long moment. Everything is at a standstill. *Am I breathing? Is my heart pounding? What am I feeling? Am I feeling?*

Then the moment passes. "I . . . I'm kind of freaking out, I'm terrified, but . . ."

"But what?"

"I think I'm mostly relieved. I'm actually incredibly happy. I feel as though a huge weight has been lifted off my shoulders. I was right: the situation is bad. It's not just in my head. Dr. Spetzler believes me; he doesn't think I'm faking it. Dr. Spetzler is actually taking me seriously."

Bill opens his mouth, as if to speak, but then turns away, and I see tears in his eyes, about to spill over.

I asked Dr. Spetzler, "What are the risks?"

He ticked them off on his fingers. "Death, coma, paralysis, and anything else you can think of, because the brain controls every function in the body." He leaned forward and nodded for emphasis. "You have to look at the odds, and I'm convinced that the odds of a good outcome in your case are significantly greater than 90 percent. This is based on our experience here at Barrow. We've done hundreds of these."

"Will you perform the surgeries?"

He nodded. "I don't open and I don't close, but I'll do the surgery."

He had a lovely, warm smile.

June 2007:
No Loose Ends

IN JUNE, I ATTENDED A WARP BOARD MEETING IN
Boston.
WARP is an acronym for Weave A Real Peace, a nonprofit
networking organization whose members are dedicated to improv-
ing the quality of life of textile artisans in communities-in-need.

"I have no idea what state I'll be in after the surgeries, so
someone should take over as board liaison, just in case," I explained when everyone had gathered.

Linda nodded. "I'll do that." Linda was our newsletter editor. We'd been working together for several years, ever since I
began writing my regular column, which she'd named, "Textile
Techniques from Around the World." We'd been friends since I
first joined WARP.

I kept apologizing. "I'm sorry I'm not volunteering for my
share of the workload; I just daren't take stuff on at this point.
If all goes well, I'll roll up my sleeves and join in." I paused. "I
can't even assume that I'll be fine within a few months, so someone else may have to take over my part in organizing the annual
meeting."

Cheryl shifted. "I can't stand it. You have to stop."

I turned toward her. "Stop what?"

"Stop talking like this. I can't handle it."

I spoke softly. "But I have no choice. I have to do it this way. I don't know what's going to happen, and it'll be easier if we have everything sorted out ahead of time. It's my way of dealing with it. I think it's better to do it like this."

She sighed. "I know."

"We need to tell the kids that I may die."

Bill turned toward me, a wet plate in one hand, a dripping sponge in the other, the water still running.

He stared at me for a few seconds; then, without saying a word, he turned back toward the sink and continued washing dishes. I stood leaning against the wall for a long moment, my eyes on his back, waiting for him to clear his throat, his usual precursor to speech. When it was clear that he was going to maintain his silence, I walked past him to my computer table, which sat in a corner of the dining room.

The sound of running water and clacking dishes lasted a few more minutes. When it stopped, I heard him lumber across to the hallway and over to the sofa in the living room. He did not follow his usual route, which would have taken him past me. Instead, he took the longer way around, through the other doorway to the kitchen, down the hall, and then into the living room. I glanced into the living room, toward the sofa, a few yards away from me; he was settling down for a nap, the sofa springs squeaking, his back to me. I returned to my computer. A couple of minutes later, I heard loud snoring.

I have always tried to address my kids' fears candidly, without dismissing their anxieties and without adding to their concerns.

Starting when Sarah was a toddler, she expressed her fear that I would die. She often had nightmares about it. Whenever she asked me whether I was going to die, my response was always the same: "I'm not planning to anytime soon."

I didn't want to make any promises I would not be able to keep.

At first when all hell broke loose, my world shrank down on me. My universe included me, the bloody brain, and very little else. Though at some level I was aware of its continued importance, parenting was no longer at the top of my list of priorities.

Neurological issues prevented me from participating in the kids' activities. I was too exhausted to go shopping with Sarah or to attend her softball games, dragon boating with Daniel was no longer an option, and watching movies with both of them in the evenings became a rarity. Extreme fatigue ruled my life.

During those first few weeks after my initial visit to the ER, I was taking one step at a time, one day at a time. I was capable of addressing only immediate issues and conceiving immediate solutions. I couldn't think beyond following my raw instincts as a mother to protect my children: I didn't want them to worry.

I was incapable of seeing the bigger picture, of seeking ways to alleviate their misery while continuing to follow my philosophy of encouraging open communication and fostering trust.

If my life hadn't been so focused on my own troubles, I would have been honest and open. I continued being honest with them, but I was not open. I walked in fear of questions. I was terrified of answers.

I couldn't hide much from them. They'd watched in silence every time I was rushed to the ER. They'd seen me having trouble with my balance, and they'd witnessed some seizure-like episodes.

They knew about the angiomas. I addressed their few questions candidly, but I volunteered little to no information.

In early June, the plans for me to have surgery in August were under way, and I was talking about it openly. To everyone except the kids.

I spoke to my dragon-boat teammate Joyce about keeping an eye out for Daniel if anything went wrong. Joyce and I had known each other for ages; we'd become good friends through our shared enthusiasm for dragon-boating. I would trust her with my life—and I trusted her with Daniel, who was also an avid dragon-boater.

"I'll make sure that he always has a ride to and from dragon-boat practice," she assured me.

"Thanks, but I also need to know that he'll have someone to turn to, someone he feels good with, if I don't come back me, or if I don't come back at all."

She glared at me. "Don't talk like that. You'll be fine."

I nodded. "I probably will be okay, but just in case . . ."

"I'll always be there for him."

Joyce was not the one for Sarah; they didn't really get along.

I needed to find a kindred spirit to act as Sarah's safety net—someone she clicked with; someone who could goof around with her yet also listen to her; someone caring, supportive, and mature. Margaret, a mom from Sarah's softball team, was the obvious choice.

At one of the games, while the girls were waiting for their turn at bat, I pulled Margaret aside. "Will you be there for Sarah if things don't go well for me in Phoenix?"

"Of course. But you'll be back. There's no stopping you."

But I still hadn't talked to the kids.

A couple of weeks before the surgeries, I was lying in bed, waking up from a nap. I lay there for a while, letting my thoughts drift. If someone had asked me what I was thinking about, I would have had no answer. Then a coherent thought rooted itself firmly, not to be ignored. *It's time. It's time to talk to the kids.*

I got out of bed and went to the bathroom. I splashed water on my face, dried it, looked at myself in the mirror, took a deep breath, walked over to Sarah's room, and knocked on the door.

"What?"

I put my mouth closer to the door. "Can you please come downstairs to the family room? I want to talk to you and Daniel about something. It's important."

I could almost hear her rolling her eyes. "All right."

I went downstairs and poked my head through the doorway to the basement. Daniel was down there, playing video games. "Daniel!" I had to raise my voice to be heard over the music.

"What?"

"Can you please come up here? I need to talk to you and Sarah."

"Coming! I'm just going to save."

I went into the family room and perched on the edge of one of the sofas.

Bill had been in the kitchen when I had come downstairs. The doorway to the basement was located between the kitchen and the family room. By the time I had turned away from calling Daniel, Bill had disappeared into the living room.

Daniel bounded up the stairs, but by the time he reached the top, he had audibly slowed down, and as he entered the room, he was moving hesitantly. Just then Sarah sauntered in, but as soon as she caught sight of Daniel, she sped up, hurrying to plop herself down right next to me on the sofa. Daniel paused until she was seated and then moved to sit on the other sofa.

They both looked at me expectantly, sitting on the edge of their seats. I turned sideways to face them. We were silent as I situated myself.

"There's no easy way of saying this, so I'm just going to come out with it."

They stared at me.

"You know that I'll be going in for brain surgery in a couple of weeks in order to take care of the angiomas that have bled. According to the neurosurgeon, Dr. Spetzler, if they are not removed, they may bleed again, and I could die."

Although we never spoke of it, I was sure that both kids were fully aware that my life was at stake. I was concerned that they assumed that the surgeries would be a miracle cure, that they would end the nightmare, like throwing a switch.

"So the surgeries, if all goes well, should make things better in the long run. But there is a chance that they won't go well." I shifted. "I could end up dead or brain damaged. There are no guarantees."

There was no more to be said. We sat in silence, staring at each other. There were no snoring sounds coming from the living room.

After a long moment, Sarah straightened her back and the corners of her mouth twitched. "You mean that you may end up drooling and running into trees?"

Her words snapped the world back in place.

I grinned. "That's me: drooling and running into trees." Then I closed my eyes and attempted to bring my index finger around to touch the tip of my nose but poked myself in the eye instead.

We all dissolved into relieved laughter.

August 2007:
Phoenix

D EAD MAN WALKING.

The sentence played over and over in my head as we walked into the hospital. Did I say it out loud? Probably not. If Jonathan, my older brother, had been the only one with me, I might have. But with Bill there . . .

Phoenix, August 8, 2007. Was it around 4:00 a.m. or 5:00 a.m.? I'm not sure, but I do remember marveling at how tolerable the temperature was, compared with the Arizona oven of the previous afternoon. I also remember noticing that I wasn't exhausted, despite having slept very little that night.

I don't remember entering the hospital lobby. My next memory is of waking up in the recovery room.

One down, one to go.

I'd just woken up from my first brain surgery, where they'd removed a golf ball-size angioma from my right parietal lobe. I took inventory of myself. I felt fine, I was thinking clearly, I remembered who I was, where I was, and why.

That was easy.

My next concern was how to greet Mum, Bill, and Jonathan when they trooped in to see me in the recovery room. Should I reassure them with a smile, or should I mess with them? It all depended on who approached me first.

Jonathan was a couple of steps ahead of the others.

I tried to look puzzled. "Who the hell are you?"

But I couldn't suppress my grin. It came bursting out before I finished the question.

Bill, having witnessed nurses and doctors putting me through my neurological paces, asked, "Who is the president?"

"Jared Cohon."

Jonathan and my mother exchanged puzzled looks, but Bill smiled and nodded. Jared Cohon was the president of Carnegie Mellon University, where both Bill and I taught.

I switched gears to address my main concern: "Am I still on for the day after tomorrow?"

Since the brain stem is the highway of the nervous system, my second surgery, to remove the angioma from my brain stem, was much riskier than the surgery I'd just undergone. I was terrified of losing any semblance of independence, or even worse, of losing my self, me.

On the other hand, by doing nothing, I was risking additional bleeds, which could also be costly. In order to give myself a chance to reclaim my life, the surgery had to be done. I was anxious to get it over with. If I didn't do it now, it would be six weeks before it could be rescheduled. My mind recoiled at the thought of having to wait that long.

Dr. Spetzler stopped by on his rounds that evening. "Do you feel up to going through with your second surgery?"

I nodded. "I'm ready."

He smiled and patted my leg. "Then it's a go."

I resumed breathing.

My head is jerking sideways. *That's odd.* It does it again and again. *What the—*

I hear animal noises, grunts. *Mine?*

Cindy's voice reaches me from far away. "Deb? Deb! Are you okay? What's going on? Are you having a seizure?"

Is this a seizure? It is *a seizure! An honest-to-goodness grand mal seizure. And I'm drooling. Yech!*

I want to respond to Cindy, but I can't. I want the jerking to stop, but it's out of my control. I should be able to stop it. Why can't I stop it?

"Can you hang up the phone? I'll call the nurses' station."

Brian, the nurse assigned to me and the patient next door, is watching me through the window. *He'll see me; he'll help.* But Brian continues staring directly at me, unmoving. *Can't he see I'm in trouble? How can he not see?*

Each time my head jerks back toward the phone, I notice it in my hand. Why is it in my hand?

And then it's over, as if it never happened. The only remaining evidence is the thick saliva oozing down my chin and the big patch of mucus on the front of my gown.

My first concern is whether Dr. Spetzler will cancel the brain stem surgery when he hears about the seizure. At that thought, I start swearing repeatedly into the phone. When I pause to take a breath, Cindy suggests that I press the call button to report the seizure.

Nurses swarm in, but when they ask me about it, they seem skeptical, until I show them my saliva-soaked gown.

The EEG shows abnormal electrical activity, but the second surgery is still on.

The first surgery took only four and a half hours; the second, much more complex, took six.

Forewarned by the surgeons, the anesthetists gave me a stronger cocktail than they did the first time around.

The ceiling was folding up, origami-style, into a smaller and smaller piece. *Will it drag the whole room with it? How will I fit? Will I become small? Will I fit inside the folds? Should I worry?*

Someone asked, "How are you feeling?"

Not sure how to describe my experience, I replied, "Everything is getting very small."

One of the walls started disintegrating slowly, its texture like sand. Sand was accumulating on the floor.

Oh! These are hallucinations! Cool.

I relaxed, prepared to enjoy the show.

As the wall disintegrated and the inner layers became exposed, a wave of the inner maroon spread across the original taupe of the wall, causing a gradual color transformation. I followed the sand's slow journey to the floor, which was undergoing a more complex color change, alternating between maroon and taupe, at first in waves, then in spirals.

It took me a good twenty-four hours to recover from the anesthesia. Jonathan told me that when they first came in to see me in the recovery room, I was out of it. And later, back in the ICU, as I regained awareness, I became agitated, or, as he put it, I was in a foul mood. Mum concurred.

I suffered from severe vertigo, nausea, and headaches. Between my blurry vision, double vision, and muffled hearing, signals coming in from my surroundings were difficult to manage, let alone decipher. When I tried to talk, I slurred my speech. *Great—now not only will I walk like a drunk, I'm also going to talk like one. I'll never pass a sobriety test.*

My timeline was all over the place. I had no notion of what happened when; everything was completely mixed up in my mind. I lost all perception of time; I could not distinguish between seconds, minutes, and hours, and, a couple of times, even days. My memory was affected as well; I couldn't remember things from one sentence to the next.

I felt as if someone or something had taken over my body. The person inside me was a total stranger. Nothing felt right. Nothing worked right.

Nurses kept popping into my room to hand me the phone. I was within hours of brain surgery, and I was answering the phone. There were several calls from Israel: Dad; my younger brother, Simon; and my younger sister, Rachel. Uncle Michael phoned from England. They had difficulties understanding me, and I had trouble hearing and understanding them.

The button to accept and end phone calls was one and the same. The surgery had also wreaked havoc on my manual dexterity, and when I'd try to answer the phone, I'd more often than not press the button twice and lose the call. In order to make phone calls, I had to use a calling card, which meant pressing a lot of buttons—and making numerous mistakes.

Frustrated, I tried to use the speed dial on my cell phone, but a nurse reprimanded me. Cell phones interfered with the monitors.

Mum, oblivious to the reprimands, was on her cell phone to the entire world, talk, talk, talking, and as she talked, she paced to and fro, in my room, outside in the hallway, and back again, back and forth.

Monitors beeping. Every time a monitor beeped, Mum freaked out and ran to get a nurse.

Everything happening too fast. No time to process anything.

Doctors and nurses coming and going. Lots of questions, expecting answers.

"What is your name?"

"Do you know where you are?"

"What day is it?"

"What year is it?"

"Who is the president?"

"Can you show me two fingers?"

Then, "Follow my finger" and, "Squeeze my fingers."

Too much noise, too much light, too much motion, too many doctors and nurses and blood tests. Always blood tests.

"I'm here to take your vitals."

"Here are your meds."

"I'm here to check your incisions."

I couldn't rest. The incisions hurt, and no position was comfortable.

"Time to eat."

I couldn't eat. A spoonful filled me up.

"Time for a sponge bath."

"Time for a walk."

Everything was so hard. Everything hurt. Everything felt awkward.

And so much pain.

Probably overdosing on any of the meds would work, but I should go with a sure thing. Pain meds are my best bet.

I'm lying in bed the day after my brain stem surgery, feeling worse than I've ever felt. I don't fit inside myself. Everywhere is discomfort; everywhere is pain. My head is exploding. I hear someone groaning and realize it's me. I'm writhing in pain, but the motion intensifies it. I don't know what to do with myself. There is nothing I can do. My body is not my own.

When the nurse finally shows up with pain meds, she hands the little cup to me. "Here you go. They should take effect quickly."

I gulp the pills and down them with the water she offers. I whisper, "Thanks."

"I'll turn the light off. Maybe try to get some sleep."

I lean back against the pillow, trying to relax, hoping that'll help the pills take effect more quickly. My muscles are so tense. *Let go. Loosen up. Rest.*

I lie in bed, motionless. The room is quiet. No one is talking at me; no phone calls, no nurses, no doctors. I am so tired, so very tired.

I lose track of time and doze.

At some point, still drowsy, I realize that the headache has eased up somewhat; it is no longer my universe. I take stock of my situation. I've had a headache since I woke up from surgery yesterday. Most of the time it's bearable, but every few hours it explodes and becomes all-consuming.

I am in pain, I can't think, I can't communicate, I am surrounded by chaos. I can't go on like this. If at least I knew that it would get better soon . . . It has to get better soon. This can't go on. Can it? This can't be the way it'll always be! I can't do this—I can't be like this forever! This is not a life.

The thought of being totally dependent on other people for the rest of my life is intolerable.

Think. Think. There has to be a solution. There has to be something I can do. Think. But thinking is so hard; my thoughts are sluggish, and the pain distracts me constantly. *But I can't just sit back and wait for a miracle.* I sink into the pillow, trying to relax, to ease the tension out of my muscles, to clear my mind. I readjust the position of my head, my incisions still raw, still painful.

Maybe I will feel better soon. Did I feel worse yesterday? I don't think so . . . I didn't feel good, but I definitely feel worse today, much worse. How bad will it get?

Tears well up. *Even if it doesn't get worse with time, even if it just doesn't get better, if it stays like this, or close to this . . . I can't live like this. Not just for me, but also for the kids. They shouldn't have to live their lives with me always there, a burden, a weight dragging them down. No. It's not right to mess up their lives.*

I swallow. *I have to do something. I don't have any choice.* I think it through. *I'm fairly limited in what I can do, so there really are only two options. I could ask someone to help. No. It wouldn't be fair. I can't do that to anyone. It'll have to be an overdose.*

The easiest would be antiseizure or blood pressure meds, since I brought some with me. But who knows what can happen if I overdose on those? I could end up in worse shape than I am now. I wish I had access to the internet.

It'll have to be pain meds; the ones they're giving me must be strong. They should do the trick. But how can I get enough? How much is enough to do the job properly? I have only one shot at this. I don't want to blow it.

I'll have to ask for pain meds more frequently than I really need them.

But the nurse stays while I take them. They always bring two pain pills. So I'll have to take one and somehow hide the other. I probably won't be able to do it each time. It could take weeks. How much time do I have?

I'm tired. I can't think anymore. I decide to rest for a while. *I'll figure it out. Later.*

I doze off.

I wake up to the sound of the nurse approaching. "It's time to take your vitals."

I sigh and reach for the thermometer. She checks my blood pressure and pulse. "Your blood pressure is still pretty low. We're going to discontinue the blood pressure meds until it goes up a bit."

She folds the cuff. "How's your head doing now?"

"It's a lot better, thanks."

"Is the incision bothering you?"

I shift cautiously. "No. As long as I'm careful about it."

She pushes her cart in front of her as she leaves the room. "I'll be in with your meds shortly."

I lean back into my pillow. I feel raw, from the inside out, starting with my head. Everything feels so wrong. It feels like I'm not in sync with my body.

I'll give it a couple of weeks, maybe three. If I wait much longer, who knows what shape I'll be in? I may not be able to take care of it myself. In the meantime, I'll start collecting pain pills.

My headache is escalating again, fast becoming unbearable. I press the call button.

I'll need both pills. I'll start collecting tomorrow.

On the following day, I fit inside myself much better. I still feel achy and uncomfortable, but the headaches aren't quite as consuming, the incisions not quite as raw. The world has slowed down to some extent, and I start making sense of it.

My sister, Rachel sounded frantic over the phone. "Cindy says you want to kill yourself."

"What are you talking about?"

"She said that you've been thinking about suicide."

I had no idea where that came from, but I knew that I should reassure her. "I'm fine now. Don't be silly—of course I wouldn't commit suicide. I don't have it in me."

Later, on the phone to Cindy, I asked her about it. She assured me that I had talked about suicide. A vague recollection surfaced.

"Oh yeah. That was yesterday, when I was feeling lousy. I feel fine now. So there's nothing to worry about."

I was feeling fine. Therefore, everything was fine, everything had been fine, and everything would be fine.

On the third day after the brain stem surgery, I was moved from the ICU to the floor.

"You're doing great. You can go home tomorrow if you want."

My mother and I stared open-mouthed at the neurosurgery resident. Time stood still.

As time caught up with itself, so did my mind. *I'm not ready. I can't.* It had been only what? Two or three days since the brain stem surgery? *I can't. I'm not ready. I can't do it. They can't do this to me.*

As my neurons warmed up, my panic increased. *I'm still slurring. And my balance . . . I can't walk to the door. I can't walk to the elevator. I can't go home like this. I can't manage in a hotel. I can't deal with an airport. I can't get out of bed without help. I can't face the world.*

Horrified, I looked at Mum, my mouth opening and closing, eyes huge and pleading. And Mum shifted into warrior mode. Her face turned red, and her eyes hardened. She took a step toward him, her motions stiff, almost jerky. "That's ridiculous! She can't possibly go home like this! She's not ready for it! She can barely stand up, let alone walk. She can't leave like this. She's going to need significant rehab before she's ready."

The resident almost stumbled back at Mum's onslaught. When he recovered his composure, he reluctantly admitted that inpatient rehab might be a possibility, and then he retreated hastily from the room.

Mum fumed and sputtered. "This is ridiculous! How can they possibly discharge you like this? It's irresponsible! I'm going to talk to that nurse. There's got to be something we can do. This is absurd!"

She went to the nurses' station and came back with the head nurse. She filled her in on this latest development, fuming yet rational. Forcing herself to sound calm, she presented a compelling case and had the nurse's full attention. By the time she had finished speaking her piece, the head nurse was also fired up and ready to do battle. She strode off to set the wheels in motion.

Physical therapists and a rehab nurse practitioner evaluated me, and all agreed that inpatient rehab was the right course of action. My case manager argued over the phone with my health insurance company, filled out the voluminous paperwork, and faxed it over to Pennsylvania. She spent the next couple of days jumping through the necessary hoops and leaping over the required hurdles. While battling the insurance company, she also searched for available beds in nearby inpatient rehab facilities.

After two days of intense fighting, my case manager, a tall woman with regal bearing, entered my room wearing a triumphant smile. Not only had the health insurance finally come through, but that morning a bed had become available right there at the neuro-rehab center on the hospital grounds.

Within a couple of hours, we were on our way to inpatient rehab—I on my gurney, surrounded with my stuff, and Mum alongside, pushing my walker.

chapter nine

August 2007:
First Steps

REHAB WOULD UNDO ALL THE DAMAGE THE SURGERIES had caused.

It would correct my vision, restore my balance, patch up my memory, and repair my hearing. It would untangle the chaos and confusion.

Rehab would solve all my problems.

Since the surgeries, I'd been completely focused on myself. Swamped by pain, I lived in the moment, merely reacting to my surroundings, without really engaging. Everything outside the pain was irrelevant and barely registered.

Doctors and nurses rushed in and out of existence. Bill and Jonathan had come and gone. Mum had been my one constant, always there, since the beginning. Yet she, too, was on the periphery, part of the world beyond my pain.

My emotions were merely fleeting responses to immediate stimuli: frustration at my inability to answer a phone, relief at a lull in the chaos around me. Even my euphoria was ignited by the celebratory atmosphere in my hospital room, not because of the cause for it—the news that I was admitted to rehab—but because everyone around me was celebrating.

About an hour after Mum and I made our entrance into the rehab center, Cindy arrived for a three-day visit. Mum took off for the hotel, leaving Cindy with me.

Having Cindy by my side snapped me out of myself. She reminded me that there was a world beyond my existence in the hospital, and that I was a part of it. With Cindy there, I knew rehab would help me rejoin the human race.

I was giddy the rest of the day, radiating optimism, prattling away at Cindy.

Cindy brought the outside world back to me—and took it away again when visiting hours were over. The hotel where she and Mum were staying might as well have been a different planet.

Loneliness engulfed me.

I lay in my new bed in rehab, soaking my pillow with tears. The tissue box was fast emptying as I wiped my nose silently, trying not to sniff. I didn't want anyone to hear me. I didn't want the sympathy of strangers.

But when my roommate's breathing became even and all the sounds from beyond our room faded, I felt completely forsaken. No one within sight, within hearing, knew of me and my despair. I was alone in this place. I was alone in the world, in the universe. Bereft. The dam broke, and with it my silence. Chest heaving, shoulders shaking, I wept convulsively, my breathing ragged and noisy.

Lonely or not, I couldn't afford the luxury of panicking or wallowing. It hadn't been easy to get a bed in the center. Mum, the head nurse, my case manager, and the rehab nurse practitioner had all gone out on a limb for me. I couldn't let them down.

I also knew that it was now or never. I was extremely fortunate to have the opportunity for early, intense rehab. Early rehab makes a huge difference in the rewiring process—the earlier and the more intense the rehab, the better the chances of a good outcome.

Keith was my physical therapist, or PT, in the rehab center. Before beginning my therapy, he administered a Berg test to assess my balance impairment.

He pointed at a chair. "I want to see how you manage standing up from a sitting position; then walk over here, turn around, walk back to the chair, and sit down."

I focused on every motion, adjusting and readjusting my pace as I moved. If I walked too slowly, my stationary ataxia would kick in—my balance was more precarious when I wasn't moving. But I had to slow down at the turn to allow my brain to catch up with my movement, or I would fall victim to vertigo. I was quite proud when I accomplished the task with only a touch of the wobbles. I looked at Keith for approval. He nodded, looked at his stopwatch, and jotted something down on his clipboard. I hadn't realized he was timing me.

"Did I go too slowly? How long is it supposed to take?"

He reluctantly admitted that my pace was slower than ideal.

He also timed me as I stood in place—I lasted only a split second before my arms started flailing. I lasted no longer when he had me stand with my feet close together, or when I stood with one arm outstretched. When he asked me to close my eyes, I thought he was joking. And I never quite managed to raise my foot in the air when I was supposed to balance on the other foot.

He placed a pen on the floor in front of me and asked me to pick it up. I just looked at him and laughed. He shook his head and picked it up himself. I barely managed the next item on the list of tasks; when I turned to look behind me, I swayed danger-ously. And when I recovered, Keith asked me to turn all the way around. He had to grab me so I wouldn't fall.

My Berg test score was thirty-four out of fifty-six, which put me at medium risk for a fall.

Abby, my occupational therapist, or OT, sat down next to me and handed me the front page of a newspaper. "Here, read some-thing out loud."

I looked at her askance. She pointed. "How about this paragraph?"

Since I knew that I hadn't lost the mechanics of reading, I focused my efforts on articulating. I didn't stumble over any words, and I didn't slur. I did have to enunciate carefully a cou-ple of times, and I read somewhat more slowly than usual, but I was quite pleased with myself that I managed to put some ex-pression into it.

When I finished the paragraph, Abby asked, "So, what was it about?"

I stared at her. "Ummm . . ." I racked my brain. What was it about? I drew a blank.

"What can you tell me about it?"

I stared off into space and then shook my head.

"Why don't you try reading it again? To yourself. Take your time."

Knowing what she was looking for, I changed my approach, confident that I would succeed. I just hadn't focused on the content earlier. This time as I read, I paid close attention to the subject matter. It was pretty boring, and I had trouble concentrating. It was really boring. It was so boring that the mere fact that it was boring was distracting. I had to keep dragging my attention back to the task at hand.

I understood each word separately, but I had difficulty understanding the words strung together in the context of a sentence. I read and reread each sentence. But none of the sentences made sense. The words were completely disconnected.

"So, what can you tell me about it?"

I thought, searching my inner filing system, but couldn't find anything. I said nothing.

"What do you remember?"

This, I could handle. I remembered one or two words.

"Anything else?"

I bit my lower lip, paused, and shook my head.

"Why don't you just read this sentence? Take your time."

This time it would work. *I'll just memorize it; I'm good at memorizing. I'll just read it over several times until I know it.*

I read each word, and then I read the sentence again, and again.

I looked up. I did remember a couple of words, but I couldn't remember the sentence.

Abby leaned over. "Let's try isolating each line."

She handed me a piece of paper, positioned it so it covered all but the first line of the article, and asked me to read it. "Use your index finger to keep track of the words," she suggested. That helped; the text stopped bouncing around.

I read through the first sentence. I went back and forth, reading the first word, then the second, then both together, then the third, and back to the first, but I couldn't make the words stick together. They remained totally dissociated from one another.

This time I remembered two or three words.

I had been trying hard. I had taken my time. I had followed Abby's suggestions and directions. Why wasn't it working? I understood each word as I read it. Why couldn't I understand them in a sentence? What was I doing wrong?

Abby explained that my poor short-term memory was the main culprit—by the time I read one word, I forgot the previous one. My short attention span was aggravating the situation.

What if I can never read again?

I squashed that thought immediately.

The neuropsychologist was pregnant, due any day. She shifted uncomfortably in her chair. "What is your occupation?"

"I'm a college professor. I teach mathematics."

"Math was always my worst subject. I can't even balance my checkbook. Are you much of a reader?"

I nodded. Cindy added, "She's a voracious reader."

The neuropsychologist jotted something down on her pad. "I don't have enough time to read as much as I would like."

I nodded. "I have days like that. But I can't get to sleep without reading something, even if it's just a paragraph."

The plastic upholstery on her chair creaked as she shifted again. "I used to be like that. Have you ever had thoughts about suicide?"

I stiffened momentarily, forced myself to relax, and hesitated. Of course I didn't want to lie, but I also didn't want to raise any false alarms. "Well, not really. I don't have it in me. . . ."

Cindy, who had been reclining next to me on the bed, sat up. "Yes, she has." She turned to me, made eye contact, and held my gaze. "Yes, you have. Twice."

I'd been quite proud of myself for not denying it outright.

I'd definitely given a clear indication that there had been a minor issue that really did not bear discussing. Cindy's interruption was obviously unwarranted and inappropriate.

I dropped my eyes and fidgeted, rubbing my left thumb with my right, back and forth, back and forth.

"Tell her about it."

I was more than a little annoyed with Cindy. My answer had been adequate, hadn't it? There was no need to stir up a hornet's nest for no good reason.

But now that Cindy had created this uncomfortable situation, I had to address the issue.

I studied my hands. "Well, yes, I have thought of suicide, kind of. The first time was at home when I was feeling terrible. I wasn't really thinking of suicide. I just thought about what pills I would use if I were to commit suicide. But I really knew that I wouldn't. I don't have it in me."

Cindy wasn't going to let me off the hook. "Tell her about the other time."

I resisted the temptation to roll my eyes and sigh. I raised my head. "That was just when I was feeling awful after the brain stem surgery. I thought that if I wasn't feeling better soon, I'd commit suicide. But I'm feeling fine now." I shrugged. "I would never do it." I tilted my head toward Cindy. "After the first time, Cindy made me promise to tell her if any thought related to suicide crossed my mind again. I've kept my promise."

The neuropsychologist nodded and bent over her pad once more.

I appreciated the fact that Cindy's motivation was genuine concern on her part, but I did not appreciate the bullying, nor did I appreciate the implication that I was not trustworthy. I felt like she was undermining my credibility.

I had been trying to give the neuropsychologist a full and

honest picture of who I was. I'd have been foolish not to—after all, I wanted to give the rehab staff all the relevant information they might need to help me put the bloody brain behind me as quickly as possible. I really did not see the need to dwell on irrelevant details, and I did not want to draw the focus away from the main issue: rehab.

But Cindy had to make a big deal about the suicide issue. It could have been awkward. Luckily, the neuropsychologist seemed to agree with me and moved on, sticking to details directly relevant to my neurological issues.

"Are you having any trouble sleeping?"

I had been having trouble sleeping. She asked me a few more questions, and then excused herself and left.

My reading of her reaction was confirmed a few weeks later, when I perused her report. I was taken aback when I saw that she actually mentioned my thoughts about suicide, but in the next sentence she added that I had said that I no longer deemed it an issue.

I realized that she had just been doing her job when writing that report; she'd had no choice. I was, however, concerned about her careless wording. I could easily see someone misunderstanding it and becoming unnecessarily concerned.

Testing, testing:

- Choose the word that makes the most sense in the sentence:
  Apples _____ on trees. (fall, grow, show, bloom)

- Choose the two words that complete the analogy:
  Circle is to globe as _____ is to _____. (triangle, square, solid, cube)

- Choose the two words with the most similar meaning: mat, linoleum, floor, rug

- Write the number that logically follows:
  3, 6, 12, 24, _____

- Write the missing number:
  $16 + 7 - 29 = 5 -$ _____

- Name as many vegetables as you can.

- Name as many words as you can that begin with the letter "s."

- Spell "water" backward.

Between my daily sessions with Keith and Abby and the cognitive testing I was undergoing, every minute of every day in rehab was accounted for.

I had physical therapy twice a day to improve my balance.

I practiced walking heel to toe. I practiced walking sideways. I practiced walking backward. I practiced turning.

In order to help my balance while stationary, Keith taught me to firm my abdominal muscles and to stand with my legs shoulder width apart, my knees slightly bent.

He had me step over blocks he placed on the floor. Even though they were no higher than a couple of inches, I wobbled dangerously every time I tried to bring my foot up to step over them.

He gave me a balloon to bat around, and when I lunged for it, he was right there to catch me by the gait belt I wore around my waist.

Keith was always right there, gripping the belt, preventing a fall.

"Does this look familiar?"

I shook my head.

Abby looked around. "Did we pass that stairwell?"

"I . . . I'm not sure."

Abby took me to the main entrance of the hospital three more times, following the same route, and then walked me back to the rehab center again, retracing our steps. On the fourth time, when we reached the entrance, she stopped.

"Okay, it's your turn. It's up to you to find the way back."

I looked around. I vaguely remembered having seen my surroundings before, but I had no clue where I was in relation to the rehab center.

"Have we used these stairs before?"

I had no idea.

"How about we try these elevators?"

We got into the elevator, but I didn't know which button to press.

"We need to go up one floor."

The next time we repeated the exercise, I did a lot better, but I still needed help. I couldn't do it on my own.

Keith brought in an intern to help him during a couple of our sessions. In the first session with the intern, Keith grasped my belt while the intern and I took turns batting a balloon, not allowing it to drift to the floor. During the next session, we threw a ball back and forth as we walked forward, backward, and sideways, while Keith, holding my belt firmly, shadowed me.

Within a couple of days, my balance improved to a point

where it was bad only when I wasn't in motion—I was back to
where I had been prior to the surgeries.

Abby asked me, "Can you juggle?"

I grinned. I'd learned to juggle when I was an undergraduate student, and I usually had a set of beanbags handy. I was
pretty good with three balls and not too bad with four.

Abby handed me three shiny, red and blue beanbags. It
seemed prudent to juggle while seated, so I pushed my chair back
from the table to give myself room to manipulate the beanbags.
Holding two beanbags in my right hand and the third in my left,
I was ready to show off.

I threw one of the two from my right hand in an arc toward
my left hand; as I tossed the beanbag in my left hand to my right,
I held my left hand open, ready to receive the incoming bag.

Except that I failed to catch it.

I tried again and again, to no avail. Perhaps the problem
was that I was sitting. I stood up, turned my back to the table,
and leaned against it. But I still couldn't catch with my left hand.
I had no trouble catching with my right. In fact, I did so automatically, effortlessly, despite the distracting *thunk* the other
beanbag made as it hit the floor.

Abby's diagnosis was that my eye muscles were weak, especially my left eye. She pointed at a big clock on the wall. "Without
moving your head, follow the numbers on the clock, clockwise
and then counterclockwise, and pause for a second at each number."

I started at 12, then 1, 2, 3 . . . 11, and back to 12. Then
backward, 11, 10, 9 . . . 1, and 12. I felt the strain, especially
when I went through 7 and 8.

Abby asked another occupational therapist to work with me on my vision; it was one of his specialties. At the beginning of my next OT session, he was waiting for me in the room where I had tried to juggle. "Abby told me that you seem to be having trouble seeing the lower-left-hand quadrant of your visual field?"

I nodded.

He handed me the newspaper. "Look straight ahead at this article, without moving your head, and tell me what you see in the bottom-left-hand corner of the page."

"It's not really there. It looks like it's blank, like it doesn't exist."

It was like having a blind spot in a car. Anything entering that area disappeared from sight. If I wanted to see something that was in that quadrant, I had to look directly at it.

He stroked his chin. "I wonder what that's about."

He shrugged and asked me to read one of the articles. Hoping he would have some answers, I tried hard. I read slowly, I went over each sentence several times, trying to imprint each word on my brain, trying to imprint each sentence. I had no luck—it was like reading a list of random words, words I was incapable of memorizing.

He wondered whether part of the problem was boredom and suggested that I choose an article that captured my interest. I gazed at the paper; there was too much to choose from, too many words. Just before I was about to give up, the word "Guatemala" jumped out at me. I'd visited there just before the hemorrhages.

The paragraph-long article was about an earthquake in Guatemala. It was more interesting than the previous articles I'd attempted to read. I did better with it—instead of remembering one or two words, I was able to recall three or four.

My knitting needles felt foreign in my hands. I wasn't quite sure how to hold them. I tried to remember, tried to think it through logically, but my mind was blank.

I stared at the knitting unseeing, one needle in each hand. I felt the outermost stitch with my left thumb, and, without thinking, I found myself making a small figure eight with my right hand, poking the right needle into the outermost stitch on the left needle, pulling a loop through, and slipping the stitch off the left-hand needle. My brain might not have remembered, but my hands did.

My eyes focused on a point beyond my knitting, my hands continued moving expertly, feeling their way, stitch by stitch, row by row, as I had prior to the brain surgery, when knitting in front of the TV.

Jane Patrick. I know her. Might be interesting. I read the title of the article: SAMPLING IS THE PATH FROM A TO Z. *On the other hand, maybe not.*

I'd been leafing through the current issue of *Handwoven* magazine, searching for a short piece that would hold my interest, hoping that the other OT's theory was correct, that my inability to read was directly related to my level of interest, or boredom, for that matter.

Jane Patrick's essay caught my eye, mainly because I knew her personally. The article didn't look dauntingly long, but sampling? I hated sampling. I avoided sampling as much as I could, both in weaving and in knitting.

Perhaps Harry Potter and the Deathly Hallows *is a better choice after all*. But it was so thick, so many pages, so many words. I couldn't do it.

Still, I had to know definitively whether I could read or not. I had to try something.

I armed myself with a plain sheet of paper to isolate lines in order to help my eyes track. I was going to take it slowly, one line at a time. I wanted to give myself every possible advantage. I wanted to succeed, badly.

I settled comfortably against the pillow, positioned the piece of paper so that it covered all but the first line, and set my index finger at the ready to follow the words as I read them.

I read the first sentence and read it again, and let out my breath, only then becoming conscious that I'd been holding it. I actually understood the sentence! I pieced the words together and made meaning of them: "For most of us, weaving is a hobby." I took a deep breath and moved on to the second sentence, my finger following the words as I read them. Again, I understood the sentence: "We do not spend all our time at the loom."

My breath caught. It was happening, I was actually reading and comprehending what I was reading. *Is this it? Was it just about boredom? Will I be able to read from now on? Or am I being too optimistic? Is this just a fluke?*

I decided to reserve my judgment and continue reading. It was one thing to read a couple of sentences, but could I make meaning out of the entire paragraph? Or the entire essay?

Despite my skepticism about the subject matter, my interest grew. I even toyed with the thought of becoming more diligent about sampling.

As I became immersed in the essay, the speed at which I read increased. I had to do everything in my power to prevent failure; I had to maintain control. If I went too quickly, the words might run away with me; I might start stumbling over them. Perhaps I'd even have trouble understanding individual words. *What if I can't even read individual words? What if I have actually lost some of the mechanics?*

No, I wouldn't go there. I had to ensure success; I had to keep those words contained.

Every so often, I deliberately slowed down. But if I read too slowly, one word at a time, I couldn't retain the memory of each word in order to connect it within a sentence.

As I continued reading, excitement bubbled up inside me. Whenever my emotions distracted me, I took a deep breath, slowed down, and yanked my focus back to the words.

When I reached the sentence "Now you're tiptoeing into designing," the song "Tiptoe Through the Tulips" popped into my head. I tried to concentrate, but the song kept distracting me. The only information I retained was something about tiptoeing. I gave up, hoping that it wasn't crucial, that the rest of the article would make sense without that sentence.

The next sentence was very long, too long, too many words. I became overwhelmed; I couldn't pick the words apart. Every time I tried to identify distinct words, the rest came crowding in, pushing and shoving. I worked at it for a while, before I surrendered and moved to the next sentence.

"Modifying a project . . ." made no sense. I returned to the tiptoe sentence—the word "design" jumped out at me. I traced the long sentence with my finger, and the word "modify" popped out. When I combined the two words, it actually made sense. I started getting the gist of it; it was something about changing patterns a bit, deviating from the original. *Oh, like in baking, not putting in as much sugar as the recipe calls for.*

When I had trouble comprehending a sentence, I'd go back and reread it until I felt I had mastered it. Sometimes I had to reread it more than once; sometimes I had to reread the preceding sentence or the following sentence to put it in context. At times, I managed to get only a vague sense of the meaning Jane was trying to convey.

When I realized that I had one more paragraph to go, I got wound up again. I tried to rein in my growing excitement. I had to be absolutely sure before I celebrated. *Do I really understand it? Am I getting the big picture? Or just bits and pieces?*

It *was* working. I *was* retaining enough information to understand the big picture. Jane was discussing the reasons for sampling, explaining how it prevented disasters and how it could be used as a design aid.

I tried to calm down. *No celebrations until I finish the article. Not much more to go.* My emotions were so distracting that it became impossible to concentrate. I reread the first sentence in the last paragraph over and over but had no clue what it said. I just couldn't focus anymore. My excitement bubbled over.

From Jane Patrick's article, I moved on to *Harry Potter and the Deathly Hallows*. I finished it, slowly, line by line, sentence by sentence.

I had been so terrified that a door had been slammed shut forever. I'd been afraid that the books that had enriched my world since I'd learned to read as a child were completely gone from my life.

And now, once again, that door stood open.

One of the things I hated about rehab was that we, the patients, were allowed a shower only every other day. On Friday, when I got a few hours off, Cindy picked me up from rehab and took me over to the nearby hotel where Mum, Cindy, and my younger brother, Simon, were staying. I relished the opportunity to shower while I was there.

Cindy gripped my hands in hers as I stood in front of the hotel room's bathtub. "You can do it. I've got you."

I eyed it. There was no way I could lift my foot over the rim without falling. I wobbled, my ankles working hard to keep me from losing my balance.

"Go on. You can do it. Trust me."

I had tried stepping over the blocks only once, in rehab, and they had been nowhere near as tall as the side of the tub. I wasn't ready for something that high. I needed to work up to it.

"I won't let you fall."

I wanted to. I needed a shower, and I trusted her, but not as much as I trusted Keith. I knew that Keith would catch me. He was trained. He knew how. He knew my limitations. Cindy didn't.

"It's okay. Take your time."

I tried to raise my right foot. My left ankle wobbled violently. Cindy held on. "I've got you."

I put my foot back down and eyed the tub again. I tried to figure out how this could work; if I did manage to get one foot over the side and into the bath, then what? I'd be leaning sideways toward Cindy, off-balance.

"It'll be fine. I'll get into the tub with you and hold on to you the whole time."

I nodded, which brought on vertigo and compromised my balance. I kept my head still for a long moment as I clung to Cindy's hands, trying to regain my precarious equilibrium.

When I felt safer, I breathed in deeply, looked Cindy in the eye, then dropped my gaze toward the side of the bathtub and convinced my brain to raise my foot. I teetered but held. I raised my foot higher. Cindy held on. I got my foot over and down into the tub. As I moved, Cindy moved. By the time my foot was in the tub, so was hers.

"Now the other foot. We can do this."

I knew we could. I gripped her hands tightly and lifted my left foot. I brought it over the rim to join my right. Cindy followed suit.

We stood in the bath together, facing each other, my hands in hers, my grip tightening and loosening, in sync with the muscles in my arms and legs, counteracting the waves that washed through my body, sending it swaying forward and back.

And Cindy stood rock solid, anchoring my body, as her eyes, locked onto mine, anchored my mind, preventing terror from tipping me over the edge.

After visiting Cindy, Mum, and Simon at their hotel, I returned to rehab, and they all flew back to their homes.

Rehab was empty and silent. I was abandoned, isolated from the rest of the world again.

I grinned at Keith. "I bet I could do the grapevine. But you'll have to catch me when I stop."

He hesitated, then gripped my belt firmly and nodded. "Let's see."

Wearing a goofy grin, I started slowly, walking it, but quickly increased my pace until I was dancing across the floor, with Keith keeping up behind me, our motions fluid, in harmony.

When I stopped, I swayed violently, but Keith's grip held. I raised my head and realized that we'd had an audience—patients and PTs frozen, staring at us. My laughter broke the spell that bound them, and they went back to work, business as usual.

I couldn't remember the last time I'd danced the grapevine; it had certainly been before the onset of this nightmarish ordeal. I was in better shape now than I'd been at any point since the first bleed.

I stepped out of the bathroom and found my rehab caseworker sitting on the chair beside my bed, waiting for me.

She opened the folder she was holding. "I just came back from a meeting with your OT and PT. Apparently, you've progressed in leaps and bounds. You've been working hard." I smiled. "They feel that you are essentially ready to be discharged."

Her statement wiped that smile right off my face. *They what? I'm what? Discharged?*

Was I ready for the real world? A split second later, my smile returned. Yes, yes, I was.

But I was alone in Phoenix. I couldn't travel on my own. Bill and the kids would be arriving in a couple of days, on Wednesday, but today was Monday. . . .

"We believe that after one more day with us, you should be in good enough shape to go home, where you should continue with outpatient rehab. We'll discharge you after your morning sessions on Wednesday. You'll definitely be good to go by then."

In order to complete his progress report, Keith repeated the Berg test during our last session together, on Tuesday. I scored fifty-four out of fifty-six—I was at low risk for a fall.

He unfastened my gait belt and escorted me over to the nurses' station just outside the gym. "Do you have any green bands here?" He nodded toward me. "Deb's ready for one."

The green wristband gave me license to roam around the center without an escort.

Wearing my green wristband, I headed toward my room, on my own, for the first time since the day I'd arrived, almost a week before.

Testing this newfound freedom, I traipsed about, stopping here and there to chat with the nurses, beaming in response to their congratulations at having earned the green wristband.

I was ready to go home.

Or so I thought.

August 2007:
Surprise

THE SOUND OF MY ROOMMATE'S GROUSING ASSAULTED me as I entered the room. Through a gap in the curtains drawn around her bed, I saw her daughter unpacking fruit and baked goods. As usual, whenever she had an audience, my roommate was spewing a steady stream of complaints.

Not wanting to ruin my feeling of well-being over achieving my goals in rehab, I almost turned on my heel and walked right back out the door. But my PT session, combined with all the excitement over the green wristband, had tired me out. I was ready for a nap.

Unable to ignore the litany of grievances, I couldn't fall asleep. I decided to do the next best thing: to lie quietly in bed and rest. Unfortunately, my roommate's continual bellyaching scraped me raw. Every sentence, every word, every syllable rasped at my consciousness, again and again and again. I no longer felt sleepy.

Once more, I contemplated leaving the room, but I was too tired to wander around.

Determined to relax, I raised the head of my hospital bed to a reclining position, picked up my magazine from the night-stand, and then put it back down. I did the same with my book.

I tried to knit, but after a couple of stitches, I gave up. I just couldn't focus on anything.

Suddenly, a wave of overwhelming fatigue washed over me. My body felt impossibly heavy, my legs, my arms, my head. My eyelids were heavy. I fought to keep them open. This wasn't just plain exhaustion. This felt different—weighty, abrupt, like the calm before the storm. Something was very wrong.

It was a grand mal seizure.

My CSF leak was more serious than the doctors had originally perceived, but they still hoped to avoid another surgery by draining the fluid away from the site.

The leak did not heal.

Two weeks after my second surgery, a week after I earned the prized green wristband, I had my third brain surgery.

I woke up in the recovery room petrified, tears streaming down my cheeks.

The nurses kept checking on me. "Are you all right? What's wrong?"

I could not answer.

The recovery room was a huge, well-lit parking garage; the lights were too bright, too harsh. Beside every bed was a cement pillar sporting a number. Each patient bristled with tubes and wires, surrounded by alien machines and contraptions, blinking lights, tubes going in, tubes coming out, flashing screens. Nurses and doctors bustled around, doing inexplicable things.

And I knew: I was broken.

Late August 2007:
On My Way Home

LESS THAN A WEEK AFTER THE THIRD SURGERY, ON THE morning of August 30, 2007, I was discharged from the hospital, directly into Bill's care. I was baffled; I'd assumed that I'd be returning to inpatient rehab. Still in the throes of extreme mental confusion, I didn't think to voice my bewilderment.

Since we weren't flying back to Pittsburgh until the next day, we went straight from the hospital to the nearby hotel. The two-minute drive from the hospital exhausted me. I was desperate for a nap, but Bill wanted to take me to the mall. Between overwhelming fatigue, vertigo, dizziness, almost nonexistent balance, an excruciating headache, and difficulty breathing, I didn't feel like braving the Arizona heat. I just wanted to stay in the hotel and take it easy. I certainly did not want to wander around the mall, but Bill was insistent. A nap, followed by a visit to the Heard Museum and its gift shop, was a compromise.

"Look at that pile of books. I'd like a husband like hers."

Startled, I turned toward the voice; it belonged to a woman waiting to pay for her purchases. She was eyeing the books I had placed on the counter before I returned to perusing the rest of the volumes in the gift shop.

Bill's voice boomed across the store. "She's just had brain surgery—three of them, actually. She just got out of the hospital today."

Out of the corner of my eye, I saw customers and cashiers alike turn toward him and then glance at me, only to look away quickly. I was mortified. In those two sentences, he stripped me of my humanity, reduced me to an object of pity, something to be tsked over, stared at, or avoided.

Someone tittered. Nervously?

One cashier said, "That's too bad."

Another mumbled, "I'm so sorry. I hope she's okay now."

My walk across the store to the cash registers was torturous. Because of my issues with balance and vertigo, I could not keep my head down to avoid eye contact. A couple of customers stepped hurriedly out of my path; another turned away as I passed the T-shirt display, and one of the cashiers suddenly realized a customer was waiting at the jewelry case farther down.

I just wanted to hide, forever.

The heat sent me reeling when the door swished open. My grip on Annabelle, my walker, tightened as I swayed and attempted to regain my balance. I had already been leaning on her heavily as I worked to overcome the jumble of confusing signals milling around in my brain.

I felt like an ill-fitting alien inside my own body. Nothing worked quite right. I had severe vertigo. My brain and my body weren't in sync.

And the pain: my head was exploding, my incision ached, and breathing sent waves of dull pain through my bruised chest.

I stood in place, waiting for my brain to catch up with my

body. When I finally regained my balance, I resumed my faltering journey through the hotel door to the outside.

When I stepped outside, my brain was slow to adjust from the air-conditioned hotel to the Arizona oven. I had to focus harder on each painful breath as I struggled to inhale the billowing heat. The trek from the hotel to the limousine, a dozen or so steps, lasted an eternity.

I poked my head into the limousine, and, with that first breath of air-conditioned air, I felt better. I let go of the walker and almost threw myself into the limo. I nestled into the seat, luxuriating in the softness. I felt no pressure on any part of my body—whichever way I leaned, the cushions yielded.

We started moving, and I settled farther into the seat, more relaxed than I'd felt since the third surgery. All my muscles were melting into the pillows around me. I was pain-free; even my headache had receded into the background. For the first time in a week, my world no longer focused on pain and discomfort; I was now able to take in my surroundings.

I looked out of the window, prepared to enjoy the scenery . . . and the world surged and swayed. I dropped my eyes to my lap, but the world kept moving. Nauseated, I closed my eyes until the world came to a halt. I cautiously opened my eyes, then immediately shut them tight.

Whenever the driver made a turn, my brain continued turning too long after the car had straightened out. When my brain finally caught up with the motion of the limo, it overcorrected, swerving too far in the opposite direction, then recorrected in the original direction. By the time my brain settled down, the driver was making another turn, and the whole process started again. My vertigo increased with each turn, and by the time we reached the airport, the slightest motion sent my brain veering in one direction, then another.

When it was time for me to disembark, the driver brought my walker over and placed it at the ready just beside the car. I waited for my brain to sort itself out before I started to move. Unfortunately, once the vertigo receded, my headache advanced to the forefront, as did the discomfort I felt as I breathed.

I kept my motions small and slow in an attempt to minimize the vertigo. I scooched my way out of the seat, inch by inch. I swung my legs out of the car in slow motion, and when my feet were planted firmly on the sidewalk, I grasped Annabelle's handles, white-knuckling my way to a standing position. By then it was clear that I wouldn't last long upright—I was on the verge of collapse: overwhelming vertigo, complete loss of spatial sense and balance, confusion, extreme muscle weakness, and debilitating fatigue guaranteed that a fall was imminent.

I stood there with a death grip on the walker, swaying, trying to penetrate the fog in my mind to evaluate my situation. I had to sit down. I scanned my surroundings incrementally, vertigo threatening to swamp my entire being if I moved my eyes too far, too fast. There was no seating in sight.

My only hope for relief and safety lay within the terminal building. Bill had already informed me that, confident the walker would suffice, he hadn't requested a wheelchair.

I had to get into the terminal. Now.

I cautiously edged the walker around, toward the entrance to the terminal. "Bill, I've got to move. I'll meet you at ticketing."

Bill had been chatting to the driver next to the open trunk. "No, no. I just need to get our stuff. I'll be right with you. Wait."

I kept going. My time was limited. Bill would take too long.

"Deb, wait! I can't let you go on your own."

I ignored Bill's entreaties. I had nothing left to generate

speech, let alone to overcome the all-invasive sounds of the car engines, the honking, the shouted good-byes.

He wouldn't know how to help, I had to do it myself, and the only course of action that came to mind was to move forward, to reach a seat before I crumpled to the ground.

I continued on my way slowly, haltingly, every step a production in itself, heading in the general direction of the door. I maneuvered my cumbersome walker through the crowds, swerving around people rushing to and fro, while trying to compensate for my continual tendency to drift to the left by overcorrecting to the right.

The only thing that kept me going was a picture in my mind of my ultimate goal: a seat, a standard airport seat, with gray, stained, and torn plastic upholstery. I was fully aware that the journey toward my goal was too far and that I would not reach it, but I preferred to do something, rather than wait helplessly for the inevitable collapse. So I aimed myself in the general direction of my target and hoped for a miracle.

As I made it past the threshold into the airport terminal, I reached the end of my endurance. I felt my muscles begin to dissolve. I literally could not take another step. I tried to hold on to the walker, but my hands were slipping off the handles. I had no voice and could not call out for help. My eyes started closing, and my breathing grew shallow. There was nothing more I could do for myself. Bill was far away, and I was going to fall.

I felt a soft nudge against the backs of my knees. I lost my grip on the walker, and I crumpled—into a wheelchair. An alert airport attendant had rolled a miracle to me just in time.

I remember nothing of the wheelchair ride from the airport terminal entrance to the departure gate. When I felt that soft nudge behind my knees and sank into the soft seat of the wheelchair, it was as if I surrendered my self and my awareness to . . . what?

I don't believe I lost consciousness, though I was there in body, but not in self. Was I slumped over? Lethargic? Probably.

At some point after arriving at the gate, I became aware of my surroundings, and by the time I boarded the plane, it was as if I were a new person. I felt like a bright-eyed meerkat popping out of its burrow, turning its head this way and that, checking out its surroundings.

I was ready for this new adventure, my trip home. All memories of the hellish ride to the airport were forgotten, all apprehension of my return to everyday life pushed aside. Nothing but the here and now existed, and the here and now was exciting.

I settled into my seat on the plane.

The man in the seat next to me asked, "What were you doing in Phoenix? Business or pleasure?"

I hesitated before I answered, "Neither business nor pleasure. I was here for brain surgery." His eyebrows shot up. "Seriously. I had brain surgery. See?" I turned and pointed to my healing incision sites.

His jaw literally dropped. He broke eye contact and shrank away from me, trying to squeeze closer to the window.

I took pity on him. "Don't worry. I don't drool or run into trees."

He laughed a bit nervously and wouldn't make eye contact.

"I've rattled you, haven't I?"

He shook his head. "No . . . yes."

"Sorry, I was kind of messing with you. I was curious to see how you would react."

He turned toward me. "Well, it's not the sort of thing you hear all the time. . . ."

I grinned. "True. It's not the sort of thing that happens all the time. At least, I hope not."

He settled back in his seat, facing me. "So, what happened? Why did you have surgery?"

I shrugged. "Oh, I had some brain hemorrhaging."

He winced. "I'm sorry to hear that. Have they fixed it?"

"I hope so, but it could happen again. There are no guarantees."

"So, how will this affect you? Do you have a job? What do you do?"

There we were, two strangers on a flight, holding an intense conversation. We talked about my fears, hopes, and dreams. His forthright questions gave me pause to think, forcing me to face some of the issues that would confront me as I rejoined the human race.

Eventually, our conversation wound down, gradually transforming into idle chitchat about nothing much, which in itself gave me hope—I didn't have to be a freak in the eyes of the world.

As we started our descent into Pittsburgh, he said, "I really enjoyed this flight. You're an interesting woman. I don't think I've ever had such an interesting conversation with anyone."

I chuckled and reminded him of his earlier reaction. He seemed embarrassed.

I shrugged. "Don't worry about it. I'm not sure how I would've reacted in your place. I'm sure I'll get similar reactions in the future. I actually thought you handled it pretty well. You gave me a chance to show you that I'm a person. I'm not sure others will."

He shook his head. "People are better than you think. They'll see you for who you are."

chapter twelve

Labor Day 2007:
Re-entry

O N THE DRIVE HOME FROM THE PITTSBURGH AIR-
port, I felt my anxieties about rejoining the human
race kick into high gear. Would the kids feel awkward
around me? Would they stay at a distance?

Whenever I return home from a trip, I come bearing gifts
for the kids. This time, I arrived empty-handed. This time, they
were content to spend the evening with me on the sofa in the
family room, watching a movie. Throughout the evening, Sarah
lay with her head in my lap while I stroked her hair. Daniel sat
on the other sofa; every so often, we turned toward each other,
made eye contact, and smiled.

Bill showed no signs of wanting to join us. Shortly after we
had walked in the door, he had disappeared into the living room
on the other side of the house, to lie on the sofa.

During those first few weeks after I returned home, I felt jet-
lagged, not quite of the world around me.

I watched everyone for reactions. *Did his eyes drop to the ground
just as I was about to make eye contact? Or was he in his own little world
the whole time? Did her gaze swerve around me as she approached? Or was
there really something behind me that caught her attention?*

What did they see? What didn't they see? Did they see me?

I felt marked, branded by my scars, my unsteady gait, my cane. I was afraid that this scarred and shaky brand defined me to the world, that it was all the world could see of me.

Bill waved his hand, pointing at the ceiling, and harrumphed loudly. I turned to see whose attention he was seeking. He harrumphed a second time and made a circular motion in the air with his index finger. A waitress serving a table across the room raised her head to glance in our direction and nodded at him in acknowledgment. After she finished taking care of everyone over there, she headed our way. Bill, intent on her progress, was oblivious to the rest of his surroundings.

Sarah whispered in my ear, "Mum, the whole time you were in the hospital, he wouldn't stop talking about the bloody brain. He told everyone. At softball games. At the mall. He told waitresses in every restaurant we went to."

Daniel leaned in. "People we didn't know. It was embarrassing."

Sarah tilted her head toward the approaching waitress. "He told her about you every time we came here."

Daniel added, "We came here a lot, and he knows I don't like pasta."

As the waitress neared us, I plastered a smile on my face.

Bill cleared his throat. "This is my wife, the one who had brain surgery. She's back home now."

The waitress smiled at me. "Welcome home. I hope you're feeling better."

Bill cleared his throat again. "She's feeling great, though she's tired a lot. Before the surgery, she sometimes took two or three naps a day. She isn't quite as tired now, but it's not easy. . . ."

He continued rambling for a while. Sarah moved closer to me. Daniel, who was sitting across from me, next to Bill, kept his head turned away from Bill. The waitress smiled and nodded, every so often stealing glances at me. I faced the waitress, my back rigid, my smile fixed, fidgeting with my napkin, wishing I were invisible.

Bill planted himself at the entrance to the main office, tilted his head toward me, and announced, beaming, "Here she is!"

There I was, Exhibit A, weaving my way down the hallway, drifting over to the left, overcorrecting and drifting to the right.

Ferna, my secretary, came up to me from behind. "Deb! It's so good to see you. How are you feeling? What are you doing here? Shouldn't you be home resting?"

I managed a hint of a smile in response. I was exhausted, but I didn't want Ferna to worry; I knew she cared.

I didn't know what I was doing there. I hadn't felt ready to go in to the office. I hadn't felt ready to face the outside world. The thought of fielding questions about my health filled me with dread, and I recoiled from the thought of seeing the pity in people's eyes.

Why had I given in to Bill? I'd told him I wasn't ready; I'd told him I wasn't feeling well. But he hadn't let up. "It'll be nice for people to see you're okay. They've all been worried. They were always asking about you."

I'd told him I was exhausted and didn't feel up to dealing with people, that I didn't want to talk about my health issues anymore.

"You're going to have to do it at some point. You might as

well bite the bullet and get it over with. It'll be good for you; you need to get out of the house. Also, there are a few things I need to see to at the office."

"I won't last long."

"We'll stay only briefly, just so you can say hi to everyone; then I'll bring you home."

I finally surrendered. I didn't have the energy to keep protesting, and his argument made some sense—I would have to go in sometime.

I sat in my office, checking my e-mail, wading through more than a month's backlog of messages. Every so often, I heard Bill's voice rebounding down the hallway. "She's doing great. She's in her office. Stop by. I'm sure she'd like to see you. Why don't you say hi to her?"

A couple of the people Bill sent over did poke their heads in briefly, though no one sat down for a chat like they used to. Did they feel uncomfortable? Were the rest afraid to face me? Were they trying to avoid me?

Despite some of the awkwardness, and despite resenting Bill for pressing me into going in to the office so soon after I returned home, I had to admit he was right. Taking the plunge was a good idea, and I was glad that I got it over with. It wasn't that bad, and having a better idea what to expect next time would make it easier. I had been afraid of facing the pity. But there was no pity at the office, only genuine concern.

Although I saw the merit in Bill's encouragement to "get back to normal" as soon as possible, I couldn't help but wonder about his true motivation. Did he associate my returning to a normal routine with an end to the nightmare? Was this his way of convincing himself that I was fine? How long would it be before he would no longer put me on display? Was talking Bill's form of therapy? Was it his way of seeking validation as a caregiver?

chapter thirteen

Fall 2007:
Lists

SYMPTOMS

seizures

balance

vertigo

neuropathy

tremors

fine motor skills

slurred speech

fatigue

blurry vision

double vision

depth perception

nystagmus

attention span

concentration

obsessive-compulsiveness

concept of time

processing speed

short-term memory

spatial memory

sequential thinking
organizational skills
sensory overload
depression

ASSESSMENTS

neurological exam (neurologist)
eye exam (neuro-ophthalmologist)
cognitive testing (neuropsychologist)
mental health assessment (psychotherapist, psychiatrist)

chapter fourteen

Fall and Winter 2007:
Rebuilding

THE SNOW SQUEAKS UNDERFOOT AS I TURN TO TAKE
in the world we are leaving behind. I move in a wide
circle, slowly, cautiously, in an attempt to prevent vertigo. I delight in inhaling the crisp air, exhaling clouds of steam
that follow me around. The receding sound of Joyce's footsteps
crunching in the snow barely registers.

I complete the turn. My breath catches, time stills, and the
rest of the world vanishes. I gaze in wonder at the hushed winter landscape. My eyes are drawn to a lone tree in sharp focus
against the backdrop of the clear blue sky. The tree is young,
tall, straight, its smooth, leafless branches stretching, reaching
for the sun. In the background, a forest of naked trees emerges
and hovers, protective, possessive, their trunks gnarled, their
branches a tangle of dry twigs.

I stand unmoving, mesmerized, until a cloud of my breath
breaks the spell. I hear Joyce's footsteps crunch closer. When she
stops beside me, I point wordlessly to the tree.

Does she see it? Would I have seen it in the past?

I am rediscovering the world. On my weekly walks with
Joyce in the nearby nature reserve, we watch for the Canada

geese, the blue jays, the red cardinals, the hawks. We track deer, rabbits, squirrels, dogs, people. Like a toddler experiences the world for the first time, I delight in my surroundings, stroking a mossy log, watching a single snowflake melt in my hand, studying my hands as I wiggle my fingers. As we move through the months, I am awestruck by the leaves changing in the fall, trees laden with soft clouds of snow in winter, the world emerging from dormancy in the spring.

It is as if the surgeries have lifted a spell that held me prisoner. Over the years of my life, I became numb to the world. The bloody brain stripped that away. Now I feel connected in a way I've never experienced before. I am one with the marvels surrounding me.

As we hike through the seasons from October to May, I become transformed, a healing of the mind and the body. During my first hike with Joyce, my steps are hesitant, my path often wavering, and Joyce stays close, ready to grab me if I lose my balance. Over time, my steps become surer, my balance less precarious, and by April, I often stride ahead, pausing occasionally to wait for Joyce to catch up.

I press the START button. The blue plate lights up with a *beep*. As I press on the blue plate, it lights up again, emitting the same *beep*. The blue plate lights up and beeps; then the red one lights up and beeps with a different note. I press the blue plate (*beep*), then the red (*beep*). The Simon responds with blue, then red, then green. I copy it: one blue, one red, one green. Next, the Simon plays one blue, one red, one green, then blue. I press one blue, one red, and hesitate. Was it green, or was it blue again? I decide on the green. Then I hesitate again. I am about to go with blue, but the machine blows a raspberry. I waited too long. I've lost the game. Again.

My neuropsychologist recommended this game to help me rewire my brain, to improve my short-term memory and sequential thinking. I haven't won a single game since I started playing it two weeks ago.

At least there are signs of improvement—I did make the correct choice this time, just not fast enough.

I try again. When I press the START button, the Simon responds with a red. I press red. Next, the red lights up twice. I follow suit. Two reds and one green. I choose correctly. The Simon reacts with two reds, one green, and a yellow. I press two reds, one green, then . . . yellow. Barely in time. My heartbeat picks up. Two reds, one green, yellow, and green. I follow with two reds, a green, yellow, and green. I sit up. Two reds, one green, yellow, and two greens. I repeat the sequence perfectly. *Beep, beep, beep*; flashing lights!

I won! I won!

"Learn something new. A musical instrument, perhaps. It'll help open up new neural pathways."

I'm not interested in learning to play a musical instrument. "How about Spanish?"

My neuropsychologist looks skeptical. "Your issues with short-term memory—"

"I grew up with three languages. I bet I could handle it."

I begin to learn Spanish.

Una cerveza, por favor.

"Dreaming. Dreaming of dancing. A slow dance. Swaying."

I'm not sure what prompted me to write those words in an e-mail to Cindy within days of my release from the hospital. The format didn't surprise me; between my headaches and my frequent disconnected thoughts, some of my writing also seemed disconnected, sometimes choppy.

As I wrote the line, I heard the rhythm in it. Without thinking, I rearranged it.

Dreaming.

Dreaming of dancing.

A slow dance. Swaying.

I reread it. It was the beginning of a poem, of sorts. *But I don't even like poetry. Except possibly haiku.* Curious, I started experimenting, adding a line here, substituting a word there, changing the punctuation.

I moved on to another poem, about the effects of the surgeries on my essence and the ongoing changes I was experiencing. I wrote others about my anger and frustration, about sadness and grief, and about the new joys I was discovering. The poems flowed fast and furious, some decent, some appalling, all of them satisfying a need inside me. The need surprised and delighted me, as did my ability to fulfill it.

"I've started writing poetry since the surgeries. It was out of the blue. I never really liked poetry before the bloody brain. How did it happen? What's going on?"

My neuropsychologist leaned back in his chair. "Well, we don't really know how it works. But in the rewiring, you unlocked a door. It happens."

I was afraid to ask my next question. "You said that in time, my brain will continue to rewire and I'll regain a lot of what I've lost. Will I lose the poetry?"

I held my breath.

My neuropsychologist shook his head. "No. Once a door is unlocked, it stays unlocked."

I exhaled, relief flowing through me.

Five times seven is thirty-five; one plus nine equals ten; eight minus five is three; seven times eight is . . . fifty-six; eight times eight is . . . I'm pretty sure it's sixty-four. Yes. It's sixty-four. Eight plus five equals . . . ummm . . . uh, thirteen. Four times eight . . . forty-eight? Twenty-four? No. It's neither. It's somewhere in between . . . Thirty-six?

According to my neuropsychologist, there's a huge disparity between the research funds pouring into the video-gaming industry and the funds raised for research on cognitive rehabilitation. As a result, there are quite a few video games on the market that outperform the programs used in rehab centers. He recommended the video game Brain Age.

Daniel bought me a Nintendo DS as a Christmas/Hanukkah present, and I purchased a variety of brain-training video games. I played Brain Age and Brain Age 2 most often. They included activities designed to improve memory, concentration, sequential thinking, and speed of thinking.

I played them over and over and over.

Sarah poked her head through the doorway. "Mum? Can you help me with my algebra homework?"

I had been dreading this moment. In the past, Sarah had occasionally come to me for help on her math homework, so I had known it was coming, but I'd hoped it wouldn't be so soon, less than a month post-surgeries.

Could I help her? I didn't know. I knew there were no guarantees that I'd be able to return to teaching mathematics. But I didn't want to know yet; I wasn't ready to find out whether I should look elsewhere for a source of income.

Sarah handed me her algebra textbook, pointing at the first problem. I took a deep breath and studied the problem. It was a word problem, something that I'd never had trouble with previously, but now I had to read through it several times, line by line, before I could make sense of it.

When I did, all the tension in my muscles melted away. Not only did I understand the problem, but I also knew how to solve it, and, moreover, I could explain it—effectively.

I turned to Sarah and proudly went through the problem sentence by sentence, translating it from words to mathematical formulas. Once we had the equation in front of us, we solved it together, without difficulty: it involved only two steps, and there were only whole numbers in sight, no fractions.

Solving the second problem also went smoothly. My breathing quickened, and my heart rate picked up. I tried to hold off on the celebrations by lingering over every deep breath and relaxing my muscles. When my heart rate slowed down, I deemed myself ready to move on to the third problem on the page.

As soon as I read the first line, I knew I was in trouble—it included fractions and decimals. Despite my misgivings, I forged on, until I realized it was far beyond my abilities—solving it would involve at least three steps.

I suggested that Sarah ask Bill for help on it.

"Bill, I really think there's a chance I won't be able to get back to teaching."

His nose stuck in a magazine, he turned the page. "I'm sure it'll be fine."

"Listen to me! Sarah asked you to help her with that algebra problem because I couldn't do it."

He said nothing.

On previous occasions, when I had tried to discuss the possibility that my days as a mathematician might be over, he pooh-poohed the idea, always with the refrain, "I'm sure you'll be fine."

Had he been belittling my anxieties? Had he not believed there were grounds for my fears? Had he not wanted to believe it? Had he thought that he was reassuring me?

Was he even listening to me?

I did not teach during my first year post-surgery. I couldn't teach; the cognitive damage was too extensive. I spent that year focusing on rehab. Once I believed that both my ability to think sequentially and my basic arithmetic skills had improved, I purchased an algebra textbook that specifically targeted students who needed to strengthen their algebra background in order to succeed in a calculus course. I planned to work my way through it chapter by chapter, problem by problem.

I wanted to get to work, I needed to get started, I knew that I would, but for some reason I could not. Was I afraid of failure? Or was I merely procrastinating? I placed the textbook in a prominent position where I'd see it every day, several times a day, as a teaser, a reminder, a burden. Finally, a couple of months or so after I bought the book, out of the blue, with no obvious impetus, I opened it, ready to get to work.

The print was large and the writing was sparse on the pages, yet I still had difficulty reading through the theory. I set the book aside but immediately picked it back up and skipped through to the exercises at the end of the section. I exhaled and relaxed; I knew how to solve the first couple of problems. I decided to change my strategy—I would work through the exercises, and only when I ran into trouble would I backtrack and read through the corresponding material.

I sailed through the first few problems and then hit a snag: I couldn't remember the quadratic formula. I leafed through the previous pages until I found it, got the nudge I needed, proceeded to solve the problem, and moved on to the next one. I made sure I understood every minute detail. I solved every example, every exercise, carefully, writing the solution down neatly, step by step, as I would write on the board in a classroom.

At first, I faltered often and had to backtrack, relearning material, reminding myself of formulas and solution techniques. There were days when I had to go back and forth between the problems and the theory, needing numerous kicks in the right direction. Sometimes I became so frustrated that I wanted to put the book down. On other days I didn't even feel like cracking it open. But I allotted myself a section a day, no excuses—and I stuck with it.

As I reopened more and more neural pathways, my progress rate increased. I continued to have trouble with multi-step problems; with my thinking speed, which I thought was much slower than it had been prior to the brain bleeds; and, often, with debilitating fatigue, which would strike without warning. Despite the difficulties and frustrations, I persisted.

When I finished working through the algebra textbook, I started on the calculus text we used in our classrooms at Carnegie Mellon University. In addition to covering more advanced material, the calculus textbook was more verbose than the algebra book and more densely printed. I had a lot more trouble reading it; a section a day was too much. I amended the rule: I had two or three days to finish a section, and at the end of each chapter I allowed myself a couple of days off.

Four or five chapters into the calculus textbook, I became bored out of my mind; I couldn't stand it any longer. I sat down, the calculus book in hand, open to the next chapter, trying to force myself to get started. It felt like . . . like when I used to study for final exams when I was a student.

When I was an undergrad, whenever I hit a point at which I got bored studying the material, I took it as a sign that my brain had hit capacity, that it was time to stop, that I was as prepared for the exam as I could be.

It was time to set the calculus textbook aside. There wasn't much more I could do; there wasn't much more I needed to do. I was ready to teach, or as ready as I could be.

chapter fifteen

Fall and Winter 2007:
Family

ARAH HESITATED AT THE DOOR, CLEARLY RELUCTANT TO leave for the bus stop.

"Do you want me to walk you to the bus?"

She nodded.

As we approached the bus stop, Sarah whispered to me, "Pretend that you insisted on walking me here."

Oblivious to any possible implications about her psychological state, I was amused at her need to maintain her image. I'd been home for only a few days; I felt that her behavior was understandable. But as the days went by, I started wondering.

During the next few months, Sarah alternated between being clingy and distancing herself.

On the one hand, she spent much of the time out of the house, hanging out with her friends at the mall and attending numerous sleepovers, and during what little time she spent at home, she often stayed in her room with her door closed, listening to music, glued to her laptop.

On the other hand, when she was at home and not closed off in her room, she sought opportunities for intimacy with me, a level of closeness she had not pursued since she'd left her toddler years behind. Several times, not only did she ask me to read her a bedtime story, a ritual we had long abandoned, but she also chose picture books, books we hadn't touched for many years.

When I sat at my desk in the dining room, working on my laptop, Sarah frequently brought her laptop over and sat down next to me, something she'd never done before the surgeries.

Usually she listened to music while wearing earbuds, but every so often she'd share them with me, one in her ear, the other in mine, our heads close together. "Mum, listen to this one. I think you'll like it."

She even listened to music she'd had little time for in the past. "Okay, it's your turn, Mum. What would you like to listen to?"

"How about some Talking Heads?"

"Sure. 'Burning Down the House'?"

When the kids were younger, we went on walks together, played outside, and read bedtime stories, but now that they were older, they were less inclined to agree with each other on the nature of joint activities. More often than not, at least one of them refused to join in and went off to find something else to do. Watching DVDs together was the only activity that seemed to hold both of their interest, provided they were able to agree on a movie. Even then, one of them often wandered away after a while.

Now, since the surgeries, watching TV together in the family room became a cherished opportunity for intimacy for all three of us, and the kids seemed willing to work harder to come to an agreement on what to watch.

Sarah would sit next to me and wrap a blanket around us. Daniel would plop down on the floor by our collection of videotapes and DVDs and call out titles that caught his interest and that he thought had a decent chance of appealing to us as well.

"*Taxi!*"

Sarah didn't hesitate. "Yes."

In the past, when Daniel and Sarah had agreed on a movie, I had also agreed, but now I had to be more selective. I vetoed any motion-heavy movies. Motion on the TV screen, whether from action or from camera work, often triggered vertigo. If movements were too abrupt or swervy, I had to look away or I'd become nauseated. I had to say no to *Taxi*.

"Lord of the Rings?"

I couldn't filter out extreme emotions any better than I could on-screen action, so I avoided movies that included scary scenes, too. "No."

"Narnia?"

Sarah hesitated. "Ummm . . . okay."

"Sure." I shrugged. It wasn't ideal motion-wise, but I could tell that if we didn't form a consensus soon, the kids would give up.

Unfortunately, tired much of the time, I frequently had to decline the kids' entreaties to watch a movie together. When I felt less than fully alert but not totally exhausted, I insisted that we watch DVDs of shows like *Scrubs*, *MASH*, and *Northern Exposure*, because they took up only short chunks of time. That way, if I got too fatigued, I usually managed to hold out until an episode was over, and the kids weren't as disappointed as they were when I had to retire to bed midmovie.

Once we agreed on a movie or a show, Sarah would rearrange and plump the cushions and tuck the blanket around the two of us more securely, and we'd both lean back and wriggle into the nest she had created. Daniel would slip the DVD into the player, hand me the remote, and either settle in on my other side or stretch out on the other sofa.

Once everyone was in place, I'd press the PLAY button, and we'd immerse ourselves in the movie.

Then Bill started joining us.

Before the bleeds, on the rare occasion, he'd lumber into the family room, toting his blanket, and stretch out on the floor in front of the TV.

The first time he did it, though surprised, we were pleased that he wanted to participate. But our pleasure quickly turned to disappointment and annoyance.

He spent a good ten minutes shifting around, during which time we couldn't see the TV screen, and once he settled in position, he started asking questions.

"So, what's this movie about?"

"A family on vacation."

"That's nice. Where are they?"

"In Paris."

"That's nice. Who's that woman?"

"Dad! We're trying to watch the movie!"

Then he fell asleep and proceeded to snore, loudly.

He finally woke up at the end and commented, "That was a good movie."

We looked at each other and chuckled.

Though he seldom joined us, he followed the same routine every time. We'd roll our eyes at each other, pause the movie while he settled down, and raise the volume to cover his snoring.

After the surgeries, what used to be a rare occurrence grew in frequency. It didn't take long before we stopped seeing the humor in his behavior and went beyond the eye rolling.

"Dad! We can't see. Get down!"

"Bill, can you please move from in front of the TV?"

And move he did. He started lying on the sofa that Daniel often occupied. Now, he didn't even feign interest in the movie; as soon as he flumped down, he rolled over and, with his back to the room and us, fell asleep.

At first, he joined us only when that sofa was free, but then he started ousting Daniel from it. He'd lumber in with his blanket, stand in front of what he now clearly considered his sofa, wordlessly point his finger at Daniel, and flick it sideways, toward the sofa where Sarah and I sat.

Within a couple of weeks, he moved his piles of magazines from the living room floor by the sofa he'd claimed years ago to the family room floor by the sofa he was now claiming as his own.

The air of easy companionship that the family room had held rapidly evaporated. It wasn't a relaxing experience to watch a movie with loud snoring in the background, all three of us squashed together on the sofa, especially when we weren't in a snuggly mood. At first, one of us would sit on the floor, but it just wasn't the same. Our initial response was to drift away; Sarah and I relocated to our respective rooms, and Daniel stationed himself in the basement.

I soon realized that my time with the kids was too important to lose. Our family was already in a state of disrepair, but all was not lost. I had to salvage what little we still had—our time together in the family room. I was determined to protect that.

"Bill, this is not your bedroom. This is our family room. You've turned the living room into your bedroom—you are not doing the same to the family room. This is for family time."

He tried ignoring me. He tried telling me that he was just resting, that he'd move later. But I was relentless.

Finally, he moved back to the living room, at least when I was downstairs. Several times, I caught him sleeping on the sofa when I emerged from my room. I had to admonish him regularly. If I found him lying on the sofa in the family room and said nothing, he stayed there.

The kids and I resumed our time together in front of the TV, but it wasn't quite the same. My constant struggle with Bill

tainted the air—what used to be a completely relaxed atmosphere now held a degree of tension that we were unable to ignore.

⌒

Daniel was having trouble sleeping, and Sarah . . . I wasn't sure
what caused Sarah's wide swings between distancing herself and
clinging to me. Given the enormity of what had happened over
the past few months, I was certain that the kids must have been
affected by it, and I felt Bill and I had neither the resources nor
the reserves to help them effectively through their difficulties.
We, and they, needed professional help.

Bill and I were sitting at the kitchen table. Bill was pecking
away at one of the two laptops in front of him, every so often
glancing over to the other laptop's screen. I was facing him, eating granola.

I waited until he paused in his typing. "I need to talk to
you."

He raised his head.

"Daniel needs help, a therapist, and, given what happened,
I think Sarah could use one as well."

His eyes slid away from me, then back to me and away
again. He cleared his throat. "They seem to be doing okay."

"No, they aren't. Daniel's having trouble at night, and you
know that his video games are an escape, and he's constantly
playing them—"

"Well, maybe Daniel could do with some therapy, but I'm
not so sure about Sarah, and you know she'll hate the idea."

"When do you see her? How many nights a week is she
home? And during the day, she's usually off with her friends.
She's hardly ever at home."

"It's not as bad as that, and I think all her friends are like that. She's thirteen."

"Maybe it is partly because she's a teenager, but I can't believe her friends are away from home as much as she is. Why doesn't she have sleepovers here? Given what happened, I'm sure it's affected her."

Bill continued arguing against Sarah's need for therapy, but I didn't let up. Eventually, he reluctantly agreed that we could discuss it with the kids.

"What about you, Bill? Perhaps you could use someone to talk to?" I sighed. "This would be hard on anyone, what we've been through."

He cleared his throat, got up, and turned toward the door, saying, "Oh, no, I'm fine. If I need anyone to talk to, I talk to people at the office. You know, Steve or Nic . . . But I'm fine."

Daniel readily agreed to see a therapist, but, as Bill predicted, Sarah objected, vehemently. Eventually, after much discussion, she reluctantly consented to give it a chance and go to three sessions, and then decide if she wanted to continue.

I told Sarah, "From what I hear about this woman, I think you'll like her. I want you to give her a real chance. But if you don't like her, we can always find someone else."

"If I don't like her, would I have to start over with counting the three appointments with someone else?"

I explained that we'd first meet the therapist together, and if she liked her, we'd start counting. If Sarah didn't like her, we'd reevaluate.

Before Sarah could change her mind, I arranged an initial appointment for us to meet the therapist.

After we sat down in the therapist's office, I explained the background to her, about the surgeries and Sarah's reluctance to go to therapy.

Bill added, "Sarah's worried about being stigmatized."

Sarah said very little.

I knew that she would benefit from therapy, provided she was willing. I realized that the chances of this working out were slim to none, but I didn't see any other way of approaching the issue. I hoped that after three appointments her choice about whether to continue would be based at least partially on fact, rather than on hearsay and on Bill's doubts.

When Sarah insisted she liked the therapist, I tried to become more hopeful, but I was not fully convinced of her sincerity, nor did I trust her seeming willingness to cooperate. Confirming my suspicions, before each session, Sarah tried to renege on her agreement.

I wasn't home when it was time for her to leave for her first solo appointment. When I saw her later that day, I asked how it had gone.

Bill cleared his throat. "Well, she didn't go. We had to cancel. She wasn't feeling well."

"When did you reschedule it for?"

He hadn't. He thought it best that I should reschedule.

The morning before her next session, Bill told me, "She really doesn't want to go. Perhaps—"

"She agreed to go three times."

"You can't force therapy on anyone; it won't work. She clearly doesn't want it."

I suggested, "Perhaps we should look into another therapist."

"I really don't think there's a point. I'm not so sure she needs it, anyway."

I knew where we were headed with this ordeal, but I held her to the agreement, partly because I continued to hope that she would wake up to the fact that she might get something out of it. After a couple of weeks, though, it became a battle of wills. I refused to back down, despite the pressure from Bill to do so.

Because of all the cancellations and lack of timely rescheduling, instead of taking three weeks to attend three sessions, it took a couple months.

After attending the promised third session, she quit.

The water in the kitchen sink is running. Bill is clacking dishes. The sound of the TV competing with rap music assaults me from the family room. Periodically, Daniel's excited voice bursts from the basement, where he is playing an online video game.

I can't think. I'm trying to answer an e-mail, but I can't think.

The dishes stop clattering, and Bill emerges from the kitchen, clearing his throat. "I was thinking. Could you reschedule your appointment Friday? I can't take you; I have to be at the office."

"I'll just take a taxi, or I can ask Joyce. Dr. Hoca's usually booked up months in advance. I've already postponed it once; I'm way past due for my annual exam."

I'm sitting in the dining room at my computer table, facing the wall right by the entrance to the kitchen. Bill is standing in the doorway between the kitchen and the dining room, his hands and feet braced against the frame as he leans in toward me.

He clears his throat again. "Oh, no, that won't be necessary. I'll figure out a way to take you. Maybe I can reschedule my meeting with the student. Perhaps he can make it to my regular office hours. I can probably do that. I can take you, but you'll have to wait for me for a few minutes before I can pick you up. I need to talk to a couple of people, and I won't be able to come get you right away. I'll do my best, but chances are you'll have to wait a bit."

Knowing Bill, I can easily see myself waiting half an hour or more. "I'll see if Joyce can pick me up."

"No, no. I'll work things out. We'll go back to the office after I pick you up."

"I'll be falling off my feet by then. I'm sure that Joyce will—"

"No, no. I'll take you home and then go back to the office. I think I'll go in early tomorrow. I have a ton of work to do: exams to grade, letters to write, and I haven't prepared for my lecture yet. I don't know when I'll be able to get everything done. I promised the students that I'd have the exams graded by the end of the business day tomorrow, and I haven't even started. I'll have to work on it tonight. It's going to be another late night . . ."

His reverberating voice invades my mind, filling it, leaving little room for anything else. Daniel is yelling. The volume on the TV is turned way up. The running water is gushing into the sink, thundering on the stainless-steel surface. The rap music pounds again and again, as if trying to drown out the rest of the cacophony. Bill's voice is relentless.

"Bill, I really need to get this e-mail out. It's urgent; it's for the summer institute." As the director of a summer program for undergraduate math majors, I am in charge of everything, including seeking funding, which I find extremely stressful and which requires my full attention.

"I just wanted to say—"

"Bill, please. I have to get this out now. If I don't do it right now, I will forget."

Bill juts out his lower lip. "Okay, okay, I'll wait a couple of minutes."

As I resume typing, I hear him make his way around me to the living room, then settle into the La-Z-Boy. I am tempted to turn around to check, but I don't want to engage with him. My neck prickles; I know he is glowering at my back. I sense his anger and animosity rolling off him like dark, stormy clouds.

Lately, the La-Z-Boy has become one of his habitual parking spots. It squats in the living room, in the corner closest to the dining room. Originally, it was positioned at an angle, facing into the living room and away from the dining room. But at some point, Bill must have rotated it slightly; now when he sits in it, he stares directly toward the computer tables in the dining room where Sarah and I often work.

He reclines in the La-Z-Boy and watches us as we type. The first couple of times, I turned toward him, only to turn back quickly after catching a glimpse of his resentful glare. Sarah noticed, too. It felt . . . predatory.

Stiff-necked, she'd whisper, "Mum, he's doing it again."

"I know, I've noticed."

"Why does he do it?"

It always cut our joint laptop sessions short. We tried to ignore him but couldn't. Within a few minutes, Sarah would leave, taking the longer route, through the kitchen, to the stairwell, rather than the shorter route, through the living room, past Bill.

His presence behind me always sent waves of discomfort up and down my back. Every so often, I would try to loosen my stiff back and neck, but I couldn't; I was totally incapable of concentrating on anything while he sat so still and ominously silent in that chair. I usually surrendered and followed Sarah. When I'd come around the corner from the kitchen into the hallway by the front door, back within Bill's line of sight, I'd feel his eyes follow me until I was midway up the stairs and out of his visual field.

DEB BRANDON

I am tempted to leave and go upstairs now. I cannot stand sitting here as if I'm his target, but I absolutely have to send off the e-mail, and I know that if I get up, I will forget. I manage to finish and send it, but I have another e-mail I need to respond to. I try to type but cannot. I feel paralyzed by his baleful presence, trapped. I have to break away; I have to escape.

I stand up abruptly. "I have to go upstairs." I come to a decision. "I'm going to start working upstairs."

I pick up my laptop.

"But, but . . . Sarah will be very unhappy."

"I can't. It's too much. It's . . . too noisy down here. I can't concentrate." I turn, laptop in hand, and head through the kitchen, toward the stairs, Bill's voice following me.

"But Sarah loves it when you work down here. . . ."

I hear a barely audible knock at the door. Through a haze of pain, I see Sarah approaching the bed. She reaches toward me—"This'll help; it helps me when I have a headache"—and places a cold, wet washcloth across my forehead.

I hear myself croak in gratitude, and she tiptoes back out, leaving the door ajar. I raise my head and gesture feebly toward the door but cannot call out to her to close it all the way. The light from the hallway slices through the crack into the darkened room and blinds me, searing my brain. My head sinks back into the pillow, and I close my eyes.

This headache did not develop gradually, like most of my headaches do. Instead, it slammed into me abruptly. One second I was headache free, and the next, my entire world was excruciating pain, reminiscent of my headaches in the hospital.

As soon as it struck, I reached for the painkillers on the

nightstand, but nothing cut through the pain, and it continued to escalate through the day. I spent the whole day in bed. When I wasn't fading in and out of uneasy sleep, my brain feeling swollen, pressing relentlessly against my skull, I was writhing as the pain sawed through my brain, the jagged teeth catching with each motion of the saw, every movement of my body increasing the pressure on the saw.

Sometime during the following night, the pain invaded my entire body. Unlike the usual, radiated pain from a severe headache, this was tangible, physical, and everywhere. It assaulted me in a multipronged attack, in all directions at once, violating every centimeter, every millimeter of my body, raw and unremitting, leaving no cell agony-free. Now, unlike yesterday, I could not tolerate even the smoothest of motions for more than a split second. Even the tiniest movement sent a surge of hurt through every cell, burning and scorching through the walls of every nucleus.

I could feel the blood pulsing in my fingers, in my toes, in my hands and feet, in my legs and arms, in my torso, in my stomach, in my lungs, in my temples, all throbbing in unison, each heartbeat adding a new layer of agony on top of the previous one.

I couldn't even twitch a finger, let alone raise my head, pick up a phone, or press a button.

I should go to the ER. This is new. It has to be a bleed. But I can't call for help; I can't dial a phone. If Bill comes in to check on me, he'll know what to do. But he probably thinks it's best to leave me alone. What if Sarah comes in? Will she realize how bad it is? What if she finds me unconscious? Or worse . . .

I did not go to the ER. Instead, I fell asleep.

I swayed in my seat. I had to lie down. I had to go to bed. I stumbled toward the stairs, first gripping my desk, then the kitchen table, then the chair, and then leaning heavily against the wall. Bill was by the front door, near the foot of the stairs, watching me. I hoped for help, but he said, "Let's go out to dinner."

I gaped at him. "I'm exhausted. I have to lie down."

"But the kids really want to go, and I could really use a break from cooking."

"Why don't you take the kids, and I'll stay home?"

"But the kids will be disappointed. They hardly get to spend time with you anymore; you're always napping. And I don't like leaving you home alone; I'll worry."

"But, Bill," I began, but I knew it was futile. "Can we at least go somewhere quiet?"

He took us to the restaurant of his choice, one of the noisiest and most crowded in the area. "Both kids really like it. There aren't many places they both like. You like it, too."

I wasn't sure that the kids were really enamored with it, and I certainly wasn't, but Bill wanted to go there. Too tired to argue, I surrendered again.

The noise was deafening. Neon lights were flashing. It was unbelievably crowded.

I balked at the door. "I can't go in there. It's too much."

Bill stood firm right behind me. I couldn't retreat.

The tables were close together, all occupied. "No tables." I turned to leave.

Bill pushed past me and pointed. "No, there's one."

"I can't."

"We're already here, and the kids are really hungry."

It was a table for two, with four chairs around it. To reach it, we squeezed between chairs, tables, diners, and waiters. I held on to the back of Daniel's shirt, and Sarah held on to my hand as we followed Bill.

We had to yell to be heard. The service was extremely slow. The kids complained about the food. Passing waiters bumped and pushed my chair. I was bombarded from all directions. I had to get out. "I'll go sit in the car."

"Oh, no—I'd feel funny about that."

I gritted my teeth and balled my hands into fists but quickly realized I couldn't have made it to the door on my own anyway. As long as the family stayed at the table, I was trapped.

By the time we got out of there, approximately two hours later, I was in extreme distress. I had become hypersensitive to any sensory input. I cringed at each streetlight we passed. Sarah was singing softly in the backseat; every note ripped into my brain.

Suddenly, awareness flashed through my mind: I needed to be home, in my room, where it was quiet, where I could recover. Up to that point, I had been reacting, knowing that I needed to get away but not truly understanding what was going on. This was the first time I was fully conscious of cause and effect: the sensory input was doing this to me, and not only did I have to get away from the worst of it, but now that I'd become hypersensitive to any form of input, I needed complete relief.

Just before the turnoff to get home, Bill announced, "I need to do some shopping."

"Bill, I have to go home. I'm in really bad shape. I can't handle anything more."

"But I'd rather not make the detour to take you home first. I'm tired, and it's getting late."

I was desperate and insisted. Bill and the kids dropped me off at the house and left for the shopping center.

On my way inside, I started crying. I sobbed my way upstairs and threw myself on the bed. I soaked the pillow through and through, howling my torment into the silence of the blessedly empty house.

After my tears dried up, I got up and paced the room for what seemed like an eternity, my head filled with incoherent thoughts. When I regained my self-awareness, I found myself wringing my hands and repeating the phrase "what to do?" over and over again.

chapter sixteen

Fall and Winter 2007: Water

L AKE IZABAL BROUGHT ME PEACE.
After a long drive from Rabinal, we arrived at the hotel
on the shore of Lake Izabal in the afternoon. Tere and
Dinah were assigned one bungalow, Samantha and I another. I
commandeered the hammock outside our bungalow while the
others wandered off to explore.

I lay in the hammock, swaying, relaxed, watching the world
go by. Three smiling dogs trotted along the shoreline, their tails
wagging. A group of boys ambled past me, carrying fishing rods.
A young couple lingered hand in hand, gazing out at the lake.

In the morning, we ate breakfast facing the water, silent. I
chewed absentmindedly, my eyes resting on the ripples.

A canoe glided by soundlessly, two fishermen paddling with
barely a splash. They disappeared behind the trees, reappeared
silently, and cast their nets like whispers across the water.

I'd been on tour with friends in Guatemala for a few days
now. In addition to giving me a break from home life and fulfill-
ing my desire to explore Guatemala, the trip also afforded me
the opportunity to investigate practical aspects of my dream job.

When I joined WARP (Weave A Real Peace) in 2001, I

dreamed of helping indigenous textile artisans earn a living wage through their textile traditions. Prior to the surgeries, I'd thought of it as a project for my retirement. But now that there was a realistic chance that I might need a career alternative to teaching, I realized that the time to pursue this new vocation might be much sooner.

Dinah, the founder of WARP, worked for a cooperative that helped Mayan weavers in Guatemala to improve their quality of life. As part of the trip, we spent a few days near Rabinal with a group of weavers while Samantha taught them a new weaving technique to increase their productivity.

After our time with the weavers, Dinah and her partner, Tere, took Samantha and me on a tour. From Rabinal we headed east to Lake Izabal; Samantha and Dinah chatted the whole way. I had been battling fatigue since I'd arrived in the country, and my sensitivity to sensory input had been increasing steadily. As we drove, Dinah's and Samantha's soft voices grew harsher and harsher to my ears, flaying my nerves to shreds.

We reached our lodging on Izabal's shore just in time to prevent a meltdown. The quiet solitude I enjoyed there began to restore me.

After too short a time—less than twenty-four hours—we continued farther east, toward the Caribbean Sea. It was dark by the time we arrived at the hotel.

We sat together at a table in the outdoor bar, my friends talking over the loud background music. I was quiet, wiped out, too tired to join in. Their chatter went on and on and quickly lost meaning. The cacophonous music invaded my entire consciousness, competing with the increasingly pervasive clamor of my friends' voices. The explosive din of the distant waves crashing against the rocks echoed the thunderous sound of my heartbeat.

I couldn't shut out the noise. No longer able to contain my distress, I stumbled away to sit by the nearby pool, where the lighting was softer and the sounds were muted to a bearable degree.

Why am I reacting like this? What's wrong with me?

Tere joined me. "Is there anything I can do to help?"

I shook my head. "No. I'm not sure. Just sit with me."

We sat in silence. I gazed at the water, mesmerized by the constant motion of the light reflected on the ripples, hypnotized by silky caresses of the water licking at my feet. My tears dried to a trickle and finally stopped altogether.

On the evening before I flew home from Guatemala, we went out to dinner with a group of friends. The restaurant was crowded and noisy, its walls adorned with brightly colored frescoes.

I weaved my way around the tables, bumping into chairs, brushing against customers, barely missing waiters. The sounds, the colors, the movement crowded in on me, leaving no space inside my mind. I felt pushed and shoved on the inside and out, squeezed from all directions. Panic-stricken, I lost direction, orientation. My eyes darted around frantically.

Where am I? Where is Brenda? And Dinah? And Tere? Where is everyone? Where's the door? I have to get out. But we're here to eat. I mustn't leave.

A lifetime later, I found our table. Brenda pulled out a chair for me. *I have to sit. I mustn't sit. If I sit down, I'll never escape. I have to leave. But where am I? Why can't I find a door? But I have to sit. But—*

I prepared to sit down, still in a state of panic. Through a film of tears, I caught sight of a door; I shoved my chair aside and bolted outside to the dimly lit courtyard, crying convulsively. Not knowing what to do with myself, I paced, wringing my hands, until I found a small waterfall leading into a narrow canal. I gazed, fascinated by the undulating liquid reflecting the light streaming out of the restaurant window. My breathing slowed down, and with it my heart rate. I continued watching the water, breathing deeply, until I was calm and ready to face the chaos indoors.

As soon as I crossed the threshold, my heart rate increased. Brenda headed me off, shaking her head. "We'll move outside, where it's quieter. I should have realized. Fredy had trouble when it was noisy and crowded." Fredy, her husband, had died of brain cancer.

When the waiters moved the table and chairs outside, Brenda arranged the seating around the table. "Deb, you should sit there, where you can see the water. Being by the water always helped Fredy."

Dinah took me aside. "You're crazy to go to the workshop. *I* can't take the chaos of the gift fair, and I'm as healthy as they come. You know how rough this trip has been on you. Chances are, you won't recover in time. You also don't know anyone there to help like you did here."

The Market Readiness Program (MRP) was an intense five-day workshop held in the Javits Convention Center in New York City, in conjunction with the New York International Gift Fair. Run by the nonprofit organization Aid to Artisans (ATA), the MRP sought to prepare international artisans for the demands and expectations of the United States market.

I paid dearly for my trip to Guatemala—a four-day excruciating headache, lousy memory, trouble accessing vocabulary,
poor balance, and severe vertigo. Three weeks wasn't enough
time to recuperate sufficiently.

But I was going to the ATA workshop anyway.

Shortly after I came to the realization that I might need to
consider a career change, I learned about the MRP. It addressed
every possible aspect of my dream job, from product development and quality control to pricing and exporting. Here was my
chance to undergo the training I needed in case I was forced out
of teaching, before I was forced out of teaching. This was my
window of opportunity.

I rushed around the convention center, sobbing wretchedly,
searching frantically for a body of water. But there was none.
Perhaps a small fountain, a pond, a little waterfall? Nothing—not even
an aquarium.

I had done well over the first couple of days of the workshop. As I'd planned in advance, I'd stayed in my hotel room in
the evenings, ordering room service, avoiding excess stimulation,
and going to bed early. But quiet evenings weren't sufficient to
overcome the intense days, and on the third day, between two of
the morning sessions, the bloody brain demanded its price. I
spiraled into a full-blown meltdown.

I paced back and forth in the hallway, sobbing. I didn't
know what to do. I was on my own. And there was no body of
water to be found.

I heard a toilet flushing. The bathroom! *I'll fill a sink with
water and gaze at it.*

I tried to filter out the din, women coming and going,

slamming doors, flushing toilets, washing hands, chatting. Still sobbing, I stood in front of a sink, filled it with water, and watched it intently. It wasn't working. Another toilet flushed. *Maybe if I stare into a toilet bowl.*

I went into a stall, stood in front of the toilet, and flushed it. As the water swirled down, I gazed at it through a haze of tears. Nothing. I flushed it again. Shoulders heaving, I tried to focus on the swirling water, then studied the stream of water as the bowl refilled. The tears did not abate. Too much background noise? I waited for a lull in the action outside my stall and flushed the toilet once more. My thoughts continued to dart around, turning every which way, leading nowhere, steering me everywhere, and I continued to cry. I sat down on the seat, my head in my hands. *Perhaps it's not the sight of the water; perhaps it's the sound.*

I tried to listen to the water running down the drain as people washed their hands, but I couldn't ignore the high heels clicking across the floor, the hand dryer blasting, and the locks snapping into place. I got up and flushed the toilet again, my tears spilling into the bowl, and tried to concentrate on watching and listening. It was no good.

I waited until there was a break in the surrounding noise, then left my stall, washed my hands, splashed cold water on my face, and walked out of the bathroom.

Blinded by my tears, I felt lost. I wandered off, first in one direction, then—after running into a large, colorful, chattering crowd—another. I found myself in a relatively quiet, empty hallway. I leaned against a wall, resting, still crying.

An elderly security guard down the hall glanced at me. I was afraid he'd try to engage me in conversation, but he looked away. A couple of minutes later, he started talking to a woman who must have been standing just around the corner, out of sight. Other than the occasional monosyllabic response from her, the guard did most of the talking.

That day I learned a new trick to soothe the soul: when there's no body of water in sight, the quiet voice of an elderly security guard droning on and on can do the job.

chapter seventeen

Fall and Winter 2007:
Discoveries

I'D BEEN ON THE PHONE TO CINDY, ALL TOO FREQUENTLY
sobbing, every day since I'd been discharged from the hospital. Two or three daily bouts of crying was the norm.

I blubbered over the numerous mistakes I made as I warped my loom, I wept over my difficulties remembering a particular knitting technique, and I cried when I was too tired to watch a movie with my kids.

Many of my tears were over trivialities that would have been mild irritants in the past: a leaky milk carton, a lost pencil, a wet towel left crumpled on the carpet.

About a month after I returned home, Cindy finally spoke up. "Your moods are all over the place. Have you talked to your therapist about it? I think you need meds."

I was shocked. The possibility of going on psychiatric medication had not occurred to me. I wasn't like my cousin whose mother died when she was ten years old, or my friend who had been suicidal at various points in his life, or my student who was bipolar—they had major issues. Whereas I . . . I'd just had brain surgery. It wasn't the same. I wasn't depressed; I just got really upset a little too easily. I was just fragile, and, given what I'd been through, that was quite understandable.

I certainly wasn't in denial over my emotional state. Even barely out of the hospital, when everything had been new and unfamiliar, I'd realized that I needed help. Not only had I been honest with myself about my extreme vulnerability, I'd even anticipated problems due to my deteriorating relationship with my husband. I'd been proactive—I'd started seeing a psychotherapist regularly within days of my return home from Arizona.

I had the situation well in hand.

I had read in a couple of books that brain injury survivors often suffer from biological depression, depression triggered by chemical imbalances caused by the brain injury. In one, I read about a patient who lamented not having gone on antidepressants sooner. Feeling fortunate that I wasn't in that bad shape, I sympathized with those who were.

I didn't need meds.

Over the next few weeks, Cindy grew more insistent. I continued to resist, telling her that I was fine, elaborating on the sources of my frustrations, explaining away my vulnerabilities, blaming really bad days on normal hormonal changes within my menstrual cycle.

But as the tears fell more frequently and flowed more freely, I had more trouble rationalizing.

I finally sank into the abyss. I spent a couple of weeks feeling desolate, hopeless. Suicide seemed like a logical solution, a way to bring an end to the misery, perhaps the only way.

Not wanting Cindy to try to talk me out of it, I broke my promise to her—I didn't tell her about my suicidal thoughts. I also kept them secret from my therapist for the same reason.

Later, when the worst was over, I kept my silence because I felt ashamed, and later still, I added guilt to the shame—I had betrayed Cindy's trust.

I tried to rationalize my lie by omission the same way I trivialized my thoughts of suicide to the neuropsychologist in inpatient rehab: I told myself that I could never really take my life, that I didn't have it in me.

But in some corner of my mind I must have known that this latest episode should not be trivialized, because within days of crawling out of the abyss, I decided to discuss antidepressants with my therapist. She agreed with Cindy: it was time to consider meds.

I was worried about drug interactions with Lamictal, my antiseizure medication. I also wanted to avoid medications that listed seizures as a possible side effect. Given my concerns, my therapist sent me to a psychiatrist who specialized in pharmaceuticals.

I wasn't sure whether there was a viable solution within my comfort zone. It never occurred to me that the answer would be straightforward: the psychiatrist suggested simply increasing my daily dose of Lamictal. Antiseizure meds not only prevent seizures but also act as mood stabilizers and are often used to combat depression and bipolar disorder.

My psychiatrist conferred with my neurologist, who, concerned about adverse reactions to the Lamictal, was firm about capping my dose at 600 milligrams per day. My psychiatrist, determining that my depression was severe, decided to increase the dose directly from 400 milligrams to 600 milligrams instead of ramping up over time in increments of 50 milligrams, which is the standard procedure.

I responded well to the increase, and all memories of my sojourn in the abyss quickly faded into oblivion. But the memory of having betrayed Cindy's trust kept niggling at me.

Unable to accept the implications of that betrayal, I shoved all thoughts related to it into the murky depths of my mind. On those rare occasions when the subject tried to trickle into my consciousness, I quickly shoved it back down.

Two years later, writing my suicide-related stories broke a hidden dam of denial. Everything came flooding to the fore-front, and with it the recognition that these were no mere "thoughts of suicide." I had been suicidal. I did "have it in me." Using that word—"suicidal"—forced me to admit that there were no guarantees: I could become suicidal in the future, a truth that shook my very foundations.

One hundred fifty-five messages over a period of three weeks, from family, friends, students, and colleagues.

A couple of days before I went into surgery, Bill set up a CarePage for me. CarePages (www.carepages.com) are free, per-sonal, private web pages that help family and friends communi-cate while a patient is ill. Bill could post updates about me on my CarePage for the many people who'd asked to be kept in the loop. Friends and family members could also post messages for me to read when I was able.

While I was in the hospital, I read through the posts a cou-ple of times. I was touched by the heartfelt messages, amused by the lighthearted ones, and puzzled by expressions of deep con-cern. Their concern didn't make sense to me; I literally couldn't understand why they were so worried.

After I returned home, Bill suggested that I read through all the messages again and copy the ones I wanted to keep. But I couldn't. I didn't want any reminders of the surgeries. I wanted to put my hospital stay behind me. I wanted to move on. Over the next few months, whenever he repeated his suggestion, I became edgy and unsettled and quickly found a distraction.

Shortly after I returned from my trip to Guatemala, Bill reminded me once more about the CarePage messages. Was that why I finally sat at my computer to read through my CarePage?

Around the same time, I started feeling as if I were awakening from a long, uneasy sleep. Perhaps now that I was managing my depression better, I was able to extend my awareness outward. Perhaps it was due to the natural healing process.

Whatever the reason, one day more than four months after I was discharged from the hospital, I found myself curious about the messages on my CarePage. I was interested in what others saw, and how they viewed my time in the hospital. I'd reached a point where I could afford the luxury of curiosity. And I believed I could be reminded of my surgeries without falling apart.

I began to read. The first few messages were from people I was on friendly terms with but barely knew, and they barely knew me.

I didn't understand. Of course, any decent human being would have reacted with sympathy to the news that I was headed for surgery, but I hadn't been aware that any of them were even aware of the surgery, let alone cared enough to send me encouraging messages.

Several mentioned that they were praying for me or sending good thoughts my way. Sure, things could have turned out worse, but prayers? Did they seriously think I could have died? There was the theoretical possibility, but . . . of course I wouldn't have died.

Then I reached the messages from my family.

August 8, 2007, 05:45 p.m. PDT

I'm so glad I made it here to see you. You are amazing! You are the only person I know whose first words after a round of brain surgery would be

"Did they say I would be ready for surgery again on Friday?" Okay, I lie. The first words were "Who on earth are you?" (So as not to scare anyone, I should add that you were joking!) I don't dare post the post-op picture I took of you when you were making funny faces for the camera.

Can't wait till this episode is over! I have this fond memory of holding your hand and walking around with you during recess at school in Geneva. Talk about a lifetime ago. Maybe this experience is reminding me of my role as the protective older brother.

Love you,

—*Jonathan*

He'd written it after the first surgery. He'd been right there in the hospital. He'd known exactly what was going on. There'd been no reason for him to be anxious. Had there? Had he really thought . . .

Simon wrote of sitting at work, staring blankly at a pile of papers, thinking of me. I had trouble imagining my little brother staring blankly at anything; I always thought of him as the most grounded of us lot.

Dad's poem also threw me:

SURVIVAL

"Life's funny." "Compared to what?"
The problem is we just don't know.
What "selfish gene" caused your angiomas
(Or mine, for that matter)?
Can medical miracles protect the kids?

Months of worry and now, sun through the cloud.
But still no way to put the clock back.
What happens next? What happened then?
Wanting for it all to be over,

But knowing it really can't be,
Still, some respite from the roller coaster,
These endless waves of hope and fear.

Time never does march on
But only staggers from side to side,
Dragging us from one "event"
To the next. But what a ride!
"It's good to be alive, as long as you survive."

As I read, my chest tightened. I clenched my jaw and swallowed repeatedly in an unsuccessful attempt to prevent tears.

After I finished reading the last of the 155 messages, I stared unseeing at the computer screen. Clearly, going in for brain surgery was a big deal, but all these people had honestly believed that I might have died under the knife. I thought back to the many hugs I'd received after I'd come home. When people, some of them almost strangers, had said, "We're glad you're alive," they had really meant it.

How could I have been so oblivious to their fears?

I blubbered over the phone to Cindy, "I had no idea how scared people were, how scared you were. I didn't know. I'm so sorry I caused all that fear. I didn't really think I was going to die—it never occurred to me that other people would think I would. I didn't get the enormity of it all."

Except that I had been aware of the possibility that I wouldn't survive the surgeries. I'd set up all those safety nets for the kids. Why had I said that to Cindy? Had I not truly believed that I might die? Was all the fear I read into the messages really there? Or was I projecting my own fear into them, a raw fear that swamped me as I relived the surgeries while rereading the CarePage?

Now, more than four years postsurgery, I reread the messages on my CarePage again. Again, my tears spill over, my shoulders shake, whimpers punctuate my ragged breathing. But I'm still not sure what name to give my emotions. Guilt? Why would I feel guilty? Fear, or vivid memories of fear? Grief? Grief over what? Grief for whom?

Shortly after I was diagnosed, in the fall of 2006, I learned that there was a chance that my condition was hereditary. I knew, in theory, that if I did indeed carry one of the defective genes that cause angiomas, there was a 50 percent chance that my kids also carried that gene. I fretted over it, but only for a short time. As long as my angiomas were asymptomatic, it was all very much in the abstract. Perhaps my condition was familial, perhaps not.

In March 2007, my cousin Kevin, a geneticist, informed me via e-mail that the number of angiomas in my brain was an indication that in my case, the disease was probably familial. The possible danger to my kids became real. I was horrified and guilt-ridden at the thought.

But, twenty-four hours after reading Kevin's e-mail, I experienced my first acute brain hemorrhage, and all hell broke loose, driving out my concerns about the children.

After my first brain bleed, during my follow-up visit to the neurologist, though I was still in shock and very much self-absorbed, my thoughts returned momentarily to the kids. I couldn't bear the thought of their suffering through a similar nightmare. I asked about having them undergo brain MRIs to determine whether they also had angiomas.

My neurologist recommended that we do so at a later date; there was no hurry, since neither Sarah nor Daniel was symptomatic. Bill and I agreed readily—I was incapable of anything beyond daily survival—and my concern for the kids retreated into hiding.

During the worst of the experience, when I was wrapped up in myself and my health problems, mothering had come in fits and starts. Gradually, as I recovered from the surgeries and my awareness spread further outward, I became more consistent in my maternal role.

About six months postsurgery, my worries about the kids' health resurfaced and stuck with me long enough that they grew into full-fledged fears. That 50 percent probability was unthinkable. The thought of the threat to their lives . . .

I had to do something.

I made appointments for them to have MRIs.

The first time I went in for an MRI, people warned me of the horror of the experience.

A friend mentioned, "I've heard it's deafening."

Mum told me, "Apparently, it's very claustrophobic, nasty."

I forget who said how difficult it was to stay still for so long.

I lay faceup inside the tunnel-like MRI machine, headphones on my ears, a cage-like device called a head coil around my skull to produce detailed images of my brain. The machine announced each scan by beeping several times and, after a brief silence, emitted a loud thumping, an intermittent knocking, a diesel engine-like roar, or a hum. Each sound corresponded to a different scan. Rock 'n' roll poured out of the earphones in an attempt to dull the scanner's noise.

The experience was anticlimactic, somewhat disappointing. Not scary or claustrophobic or unbearably loud. None of the predicted horrors.

Sarah, always nervous about medical procedures, asked if it would hurt. "No, not at all," I told her. "It's just a bit of a nuisance; you have to stay still for quite a long time, like half an hour. It's kind of boring. But you get to listen to music."

She was intrigued by the fact that she would be listening to music throughout and was distracted to some extent by contemplating her choice of radio stations.

Daniel, on the other hand, seemed to accept the news with equanimity. He just went back to his video games.

I was afraid for both of them. They both suffered from migraines. Sarah's were much more frequent than Daniel's, but Daniel's were more debilitating, putting him out of commission for several hours at a stretch.

Sarah, who'd been so nervous about the upcoming MRI, seemed almost disappointed with the experience—she chose a lousy radio station, she didn't like the music, she was bored, she got tired of lying motionless, and it wasn't scary at all.

When I asked Daniel about his experience, he merely shrugged. "It was okay."

Days later, Bill's voice reverberated through the phone. "The results of the kids' MRIs just came in."

I held my breath, waiting for the verdict.

"It's okay, Deb. Neither of them have angiomas."

I sagged as I exhaled.

"I already told the kids. Daniel's reaction was to get on the phone with a friend of his. He said, 'I'm not gonna die!'"

I hadn't realized he'd been that scared. How could I have missed it? Why hadn't Daniel said anything to me? "What about Sarah?"

"She asked whether she could still develop them."

Winter to Spring 2008:
So This Is Sensory Overload

ATTENDING DRAGON BOAT CAMP SYMBOLIZED A return to normalcy.

When we were getting ready to leave for camp earlier that morning, my excitement rippled beneath the surface of a calm demeanor, revealing itself only sporadically—my hands shook when I spread the peanut butter on our sandwiches for the day, my heart gave a lurch when I pulled my paddle out from under a pile of life jackets, and I fumbled to unlock the door when it was time to load up the car.

Despite my efforts to remain calm, as we drew closer to Lake Latonka, my rippling emotions surged into waves. As we turned into the driveway, the whitecaps of my internal turbulence assaulted the breakwaters again and again. I was having trouble differentiating between excitement, anticipation, apprehension, and fear. By the time Joyce parked the car, the waves of my emotions thundered ashore, relentless, one after the other after the other, flooding the waterfront. I was drowning in emotional overload.

I opened the car door slowly, not because I was hesitant but because I could operate only in slow motion. I watched my hand, focusing all my attention on it as I willed it to pull on the handle.

Now I needed to push the door open. Normally, I would have pulled on the handle and pushed the door open in one swift motion. But now I had to think; I had to orchestrate every step. Now that I'd pulled on the handle, I sent the signals to my hand to let go of it; I willed my muscles to rotate my arm, open my hand, extend my fingers, place my palm against the door, and push on it.

As I clambered out of the car, Joyce bustled over, carrying my camp chair. She glanced toward the squealing, chattering crowd gathering a few yards away and said, "I think you'd better stay away from the noise for now." She threw me a sharp look. "You're already in trouble, aren't you?"

I managed a slow blink. My jammed circuitry allowed fewer and fewer signals through; movements were harder to perform. She settled the chair right beside me, then guided me into it. "You stay here. Daniel and I will take care of everything."

I rested quietly, incapable of motion or speech, hidden from the rest of my teammates. When anyone drew near, Joyce distracted them and steered them away. After what seemed like a lifetime, I stirred in my seat, my circuits finally clear, my body once again my own.

Since the surgeries, I'd worked out every day on my stationary bike or my rowing machine in preparation for dragon boating. And now, finally, after eight difficult months, here I was, on opening day of dragon boat season, at camp with my team.

I wanted to join in the fun right away. I wanted to be an integral part of my team once again.

I wanted to be normal.

But I was still fragile after the patch of overload, highly sensitized to the slightest trigger. I wasn't quite ready to join everyone. I waited for Joyce. When she came to check on me, I greeted her with an embarrassed smile.

She gave me a measured look. "Are you ready? Or not quite yet?"

"I'm good." I tried to stand up, but my balance was off, as often happens when my brain acts up.

Joyce held out her arm, and together we strolled through the trees to join Mary and Marty, who were standing in a relatively secluded spot. The others were inside the house or in the backyard, near the water.

At one point, Joyce wandered off. I continued chatting with Mary and Marty. I was quite pleased with myself: I was doing well. And then a gaggle of people swarmed out of the house and caught sight of me. Mark and Pam, at the head of the group, broke into huge smiles and came over.

"Deb! It's so good to see you. You look great."

"How are you doing?"

My brain began to slow down. Before I could answer, a few more joined us.

"Deb! You made it!"

"It's wonderful to see you!"

"So, you're back for the season?"

"Is everything okay now?"

People were talking at me, expecting answers. I turned from one to the other, trying to make sense of their words, trying to think of responses. My eyes skipped from smiling face to smiling face, uncomprehending, bewildered. I was in trouble, deep trouble. My eyes darted around frantically. *I need to get out of here. But they're all so happy to see you. But I can't . . . I can't stay here. But you can't leave. It would be rude. But I have to go.*

There were people everywhere. I needed help. I needed Joyce. But I couldn't see her. Where was she? Why wasn't she back yet? Maybe Mary could help. My eyes swept across one face, then another, searching for clues, for distinguishing features, but they were all a blur of teeth and moving lips and sounds. Where was Joyce?

Suddenly, she appeared, and the blur of everything else disappeared. She held firmly on to my forearm. "Come on. Let's get you out of here."

How did I find out about sensory overload? Did I read about it? Did my neuropsychologist mention it?

Learning about sensory overload was a long process.

At first, I didn't understand why I felt as if I'd been thrown into chaos when attending a party, why it seemed as if I were entering bedlam when I crossed the threshold to a noisy restaurant, why I panicked when there was a lot going on around me. To me, these totally inexplicable, nightmarish incidents were completely random. I was incapable of making the connection between cause and effect. I wondered whether I was losing my mind.

Imagine sitting in a coffee shop talking to a friend. You listen to her intently, fully focused on the story she is telling you. You take a sip from your cup of hot chocolate. *Mmm*, it's so good. Putting your cup down, you notice the guy at the next table, surfing the internet on his laptop. A flash of color catches your eye: a woman wearing a lovely red coat has just walked through the door.

Your friend is still talking. You try to listen to her, but someone nearby has started coughing. When the coughing fit subsides, you lean in toward your friend, all your attention on her, but the two teenage girls at the table behind you are giggling.

You really want to hear your friend's story; you want to filter out everything but her voice. You sit up, take a deep breath, and try to rid your mind of the distractions. As you breathe in, you hear a slight whistling sound. You try to shift your focus from the sound of your breathing to the words flowing out of her mouth; you watch her mouth form vowels. Her lipstick is awfully red, and she's got some on her teeth.

You try once more to draw meaning from her monologue by filtering out all the other input vying for your attention.

But you can't.

More and more information is pouring in.

Though distracted, you are able to sift through the data, labeling and filing as you go. *That little girl is wearing a very pink outfit—Barbie pink. Yuck! What's that flash of light over there? Oh, just light reflected off a shiny belt buckle. Ahhh, that coffee smells good. Mmm, the yeastiness of the bread here . . . That's the sound of paper rustling, that's a car horn, and that's the hum of a laptop.* The data rush in faster and faster. The hum of the laptop is joined by the sound of fingers dancing across the keyboard, and the teenagers are growing louder and more exuberant, their giggling interrupted by bursts of uproarious laughter. One girl's laugh sounds like a donkey braying. A group of teenyboppers walks in, the door jingling shut behind them. As they pass, the sound of their footsteps trails them: high heels clicking, a pair of shearling boots shuffling, the squeaking of rubber soles. The laptop continues humming, and your friend's voice is droning. The smells intermingle. The sweet, yeasty scent mixes with the aroma of melted cheese. A man walks past, leaving a cloud of body odor that overlaps with the fog of perfume following the teenyboppers, and your friend's breath . . .

Other people have filters that help them manage all this noise and light, movement and color. You used to have filters, too, but they're damaged now. You cannot sift through the input effectively—the rate at which the data stream in is too fast. The data are piling up, clogging your neural pathways, creating traffic jams. All the sounds, sights, and smells blend together, forming a pulsating mass in constant motion, continually deforming, buckling, bulging. Random bits and pieces strike at you forcefully. When they hit, the sounds are too harsh, the colors too garish, every smell obnoxious, all movements fast and jerky. Almost as soon as they strike, they bounce away. Your brain cannot keep up; you cannot focus on anything long enough to make sense of it.

Every so often, a shape or sound converges into recognition: your friend's face, her lipstick, her voice, a particular word she has uttered. But you have no idea what to do with that information, you cannot make connections, you have lost the ability to catalog. Even if you could find your internal filing cabinets, you are incapable of performing the task of filing.

You focus on making eye contact with your friend; movement now requires your full attention. You have become hyperaware of the world without and within, of every muscle and every muscle fiber in your neck as you turn your head toward her. You can feel the wave of motion traveling across each muscle as the fibers take turns extending and contracting in order to perform the turn. You are aware of the signals as they proceed from your brain toward those muscle fibers. You follow each signal on its journey, encouraging it, cheering it on.

There's too much for your brain to handle. There is nothing to ground you; there is no frame of reference to guide you. You know that you should be doing something to sort out the mess, but you have no idea how to go about it, where to begin. Your thoughts jam up like sludge in the neck of a funnel.

Your ability to think, to act, tapers into slow motion.

You are suffering from sensory overload.

Once I had a name for it—sensory overload—my fear that I

was losing my mind receded. But though I understood the literal meaning of the name, I did not connect it with the cause.

When I first became aware of the notion of overload, the awareness didn't stay with me. I rediscovered it several times— during different conversations with my neuropsychologist, while on the phone with Cindy or my parents, and in reading material that crossed my path at various points. I just kept losing the connection between theory and reality.

It wasn't until mid-November that the connection stuck. In a noisy and crowded restaurant with Bill and the kids, I suffered one of my more memorable cases of sensory overload and subsequent meltdown. After I got back home and my brain finally returned to lucidity, it clicked. I was incredulous at the revelation that what I had just experienced was caused by the assault on my senses.

After that revelation, I finally started recognizing the symptoms for what they were. I began learning how to prevent overload by minimizing my exposure to overwhelming levels of sensory input. I cut back on attending obvious culprits, such as social gatherings and other crowded events.

Unfortunately, over the next few months, the connection between cause and effect was still sufficiently tenuous that I often missed cues and didn't recognize the danger until I was too far gone, unable to physically extricate myself.

Adding insult to injury, on some level I continued to believe that if I just tried harder, I would have more control over the situation. Why could I not recognize the symptoms before the point of no return? Why did I allow myself to reach the stage where I could not function? Why could I not prevent the meltdowns? Was I in fact seeking attention?

While I was in a state of overload, I could feel the emotional turmoil feeding into the chaos in my mind, which in turn intensified my frustrations and self-doubt. I could feel the emotional feedback loop take shape, but I could not prevent or halt it once it began. I came out of each episode frustrated and grief-stricken. I became afraid that this affliction would forever plague me, that I would never be fully independent.

More than six months after the surgeries, I came across the book *Over My Head*, by Claudia Osborn. The author suffered a brain injury as a result of an accident. Reading her book taught me that I was not alone, that most of the changes I'd been experiencing were not uncommon among brain injury survivors, that these were symptoms of a brain injury, and that these symptoms had names.

I learned that the emotional feedback loops had a name, "flooding," and that flooding is a direct consequence of overload. Naming these episodes brought the validation I needed so badly. I wasn't being melodramatic. I wasn't handling things inadequately. I was coping with a bona fide symptom.

I gained further validation several months later, after my neuropsychologist witnessed several of my episodes at dragon boat races and in his office. He had witnessed similar behavior in other patients, though mine was one of the more extreme cases.

By removing the self-doubt that had been feeding into the chaos, I achieved a minimal level of objectivity, which allowed me to improve on early detection and to begin applying some coping mechanisms. I continued to suffer from frequent bouts of overload and flooding, but now, every great once in a while, I managed to prevent an episode.

The first time I needed to use the bathroom at dragon boat camp, I wandered over to the house without thinking and opened the front door, fully intending to step inside and search for the restroom.

Several voices greeted me as soon as I popped my head in the door. Identifying a potential overload trigger and feeling the first signs of a freeze coming on, I immediately retreated, scuttling over to my chair by the car while I was still able. Several months prior to camp, I probably would have hesitated for a split second, doubting my judgment, wondering whether I was over-dramatizing or not pushing myself hard enough. That split second would have made all the difference— I would have found myself fully frozen, unable to escape on my own.

During this phase of recovery, I also learned to set up safety nets for the unavoidable situations when I expected trouble. I brought earplugs along with me or asked friends to keep an eye on me and lead me away, if necessary.

The journey toward effectively managing overload continues. Today, several years postsurgery, overload and flooding still impact my life dramatically, restricting my activities. The episodes occur less frequently, possibly because of my improved ability to take preventative measures. Occasionally, probably because of the cumulative effect of overload, they catch me by surprise.

On overload-free days, I can speak calmly about knowing that I will always have issues with it. But on bad days, I cannot accept it. How can you fully accept watching yourself descend into chaos, knowing that you'll be stuck there until help arrives?

chapter nineteen

Spring 2008:
Ready

I WALKED INTO MY NEUROLOGIST'S OFFICE APPREHENSIVE, not about the results of the MRI and the state of my health, but about whether I'd be permitted to drive.

According to Pennsylvania state law, I had to be seizure-free for six months before I'd be allowed back behind the wheel. I believed I had suffered my last seizure while in the hospital.

Bill often complained that he was overwhelmed by all the additional driving he now had to do, chauffeuring the kids around and transporting me to and from medical appointments and work.

I tried to keep my requests to a minimum: my medical appointments, trips to the office, a couple of stops at the grocery store. I rarely asked him to drive me anywhere that was not absolutely necessary.

I tried to be more independent by taking taxis. But Bill worried about the expense, so I used cabs no more than half a dozen times, when there was no other choice. I suggested that we explore a medical assistance transportation program, but Bill told me he'd already done the research and was convinced I wouldn't qualify.

My therapist, in her quest to help me gain more control over my life, gave me the name of a retiree who supplemented her income by acting as a chauffeur. I went as far as contacting her, but Bill said he felt uncomfortable about it, that we didn't know enough about the woman's driving record, so I didn't pursue it further.

I needed to drive.

According to my neurologist, the MRI results showed that the sizes of the angiomas that had bled were significantly reduced, though there was still evidence of remnants. Remnants of what? Angiomas? Hadn't they been removed?

I didn't ask, because he seemed pleased and that was good enough, and because driving was a much more pressing issue. "What about driving?"

"Have you had any episodes since the surgeries?"

I shook my head impatiently. There had been those odd episodes when I'd suddenly become totally wiped out, but they were irrelevant. He was referring to seizures.

He cleared me to drive starting March 1, 2008, six weeks away, exactly six months after my last day in the hospital, almost a year since I had last sat behind a wheel. I couldn't wait!

Once I was allowed back into the driver's seat, I could arrange my appointments at my own convenience. I could pace myself better at work and drive home before fatigue crippled me. I could shop when I felt fully alert and able, and I would no longer have to limit my activities to the absolute minimum. I could spend more time with the kids, be a better mum, taking Sarah shopping and Daniel dragon boating. I could stop by the bookstore, go to lunch with friends, drive to the nature conservancy for a walk, leave the house on a whim.

When I could drive, I would no longer be tied to Bill's schedule and choices.

"I just want to get in the boat."

Today is the first day of dragon boat season, my first since my surgeries. Every day for eight months, I have worked out, preparing myself for this day, this season. As winter has turned to spring, I have faithfully continued daily rehab and workouts. I have grown stronger, both physically and psychologically.

Thanks to my mounting excitement and the constant stream of sensory input from my exuberant teammates, I have been in a continual state of low-level overload. I need to stay away from the thick of things as long as possible to prevent triggering full-blown overload, so I sit in my camp chair among the trees, away from the hubbub, waiting.

I glance at my watch. In fifteen minutes, it will be time to line up to get in the boat. I've been checking the time every couple of minutes for the last half hour. I look at my watch yet again—twelve minutes to go. Sitting so far away from the action, I am anxious that I won't hear the call to get in the boat.

I've been waiting for this moment for what seems like an eternity; I can't wait a minute longer.

I stand up cautiously, testing my balance. It isn't perfect, but I'll manage. I don my life jacket, grab the two paddles leaning against the tree, pull Joyce's jacket off the back of her chair. Where has she wandered off to?

I head toward the dock.

I round the corner of the driveway and come to a wobbly halt. A group of women is doing yoga in the yard, between the dock and me. I sway as I stand in place, trying to assess the situation.

I can't deal with so many people, and I don't see Joyce anywhere. The thought of everyone walking past me after the yoga session threatens to elevate the overload to the next level. I have to find something to lean against as soon as possible. I also need to be out of the way when people fetch their gear for paddling. The only viable option I can see is a pole supporting the deck overlooking the lake.

It is the perfect place, quiet, out of the way, yet sufficiently close to the dock that I won't miss the call to line up. I also have a fantastic view of the water. As I gaze at the undulating image of the midmorning sun on the waves, I feel my breathing slow down, my circuits clear, my balance improve, and my muscles relax.

The call jolts me out of my calm.

As people stream past me, I lurch sideways and sway violently from side to side. I stay by my pole. I cannot manage on my own. I need Joyce.

"There you are! I've been looking for you. Oh, good—you do have my stuff." Joyce puts her life jacket on, zips it up, grabs her paddle, and holds out her arm. I totter dangerously. "Easy, easy, take your time. We're fine. Hold on tight."

We walk over to the dock to line up with the rest of the crowd. I am beside myself: I'm shaking, my heart is hammering, and I'm having trouble breathing.

Am I ready? Will I be strong enough? Will I be able to focus and follow the calls? What if my technique isn't up to it? What if I don't have enough stamina to make it through the entire practice?

My grip on Joyce's arm tightens through particularly severe bouts of rocking. "I wish they'd hurry up. I want to get on the water."

"We'll get there. Try to relax."

Finally, it's our turn to step onto the dock. Joyce takes my paddle from me and hands it to Patty, who is already in the boat.

I'm not sure how to proceed from there. I'm hanging on to Joyce tightly with my right hand. What should I do with my left? Should I face Joyce, hold on to her with both hands, and clamber into the boat backward? No, that won't work. Should I grab onto the gunwale with one hand? But it's on the same level as the dock; I'd have to bend down low. I'm not sure I can manage that without toppling over.

Joyce has also been trying to figure it out. "Why don't you sit down on the dock? I'll help you."

Mary reaches up to me from inside the boat. Firmly supported by Joyce and Mary, I lower myself to sit on the dock, my feet dangling in the boat. Joyce lets go of my right hand, and I place it on Robin's shoulder, lean into the boat, and blunder into my seat behind Robin while Mary supports my elbow. Once I'm settled in my seat, she turns to sit back down next to Robin.

I aim a triumphant grin at Patty, my seatmate. She grins back at me and holds her hand up. "High five!" We smack our hands together.

She passes me my paddle.

I sit up straight and lay the paddle across my lap at a forty-five degree angle, primed to whisk it up over the water at the call.

I'm ready.

chapter twenty

Summer 2008:
My Place

I PULL THE BOX FLAPS OPEN, TAKE A DEEP BREATH, SHIFT my weight onto my knees, and start lifting out books one by one, liberating them from their prison.

The Bone People, by Keri Hulme; *Travels with My Aunt,* by Graham Greene; *The Songlines* and *In Patagonia,* by Bruce Chatwin; *The Once and Future King,* by T. H. White; *A High Wind in Jamaica,* by Richard Hughes. I pause when I find *The Glass Bead Game,* by Hermann Hesse. I sit back on my heels and riffle through the pages. I marvel at their smoothness; they're so much whiter than I would have expected after so many years. The book must have been relatively new when I packed it away. I raise it close to my face, breathing in a touch of sweetness, a memory of the pulp that formed the paper.

I slide it reverently in between two other books on the shelf, then rummage around in the box. My other Hermann Hesse, *Siddhartha,* has to be in here as well. I open it, relieved and happy to find an old friend. The grain is rough, the pages yellowing. It is at least twenty, maybe closer to twenty-five, years old. I open to random pages and sneeze at the dust that erupts when I close it.

For thirteen years, ever since Bill, the kids, and I moved into our house, a dozen boxes of books have remained unopened, abandoned under piles of stuff. And now that I am moving out after seventeen years of marriage, I am reclaiming these unopened boxes. It is finally time to free the contents. *Borstal Boy*, by Brendan Behan—one of so many of Dad's recommendations. *Zorba the Greek*, by Nikos Kazantzakis—I can't remember how I learned of Kazantsakis. I don't think it was Dad—perhaps a friend. *Catch-22*—was that one of Jonathan's contributions to my reading repertoire, or did I stumble upon it myself? *Lost Horizon* was definitely one of Dad's suggestions for a good read. Charles Dickens, Shakespeare, Salman Rushdie—books I read while I was in high school or in college, old friends I've missed off and on during these thirteen years of confinement.

Stiff, I get up to stretch, step back, and sweep the sunlit room with my gaze. Indian textile-covered cushions are scattered across my futon, sleigh bells are hanging on the wall, a maple floor loom stands in one corner, an oak spinning wheel in another, and most of my books are on the shelves, filling my new house with their essence, my essence.

chapter twenty-one

2008:
Help? Help!

M Y BACKPACK SLIPS OFF MY SHOULDER, TAKING THE bag and my paddle down with it. *The paddle—it'll fall. Grab it!*

I can't.

I'm in full lockdown.

A malevolent entity has taken over the controls of my body, jamming up circuits, slowing down my systems, preventing signals from reaching their targets, my muscles, my vocal chords. I am frozen, incapable of motion or communication. My body is not my own.

Joyce's voice arises from within the meaningless hubbub. "I thought so—you've got that deer-caught-in-the-headlights look. Stay where you are. I'll put our stuff down and get you out of here."

I've found that when my need is evident, help always appears. But not all my brain-related problems are as obvious as overload and shutdowns. When my difficulties are not apparent, I've learned that help is always there for the asking. The problem is, I don't always know when I need help. And I can't always ask.

It had been over a month since I'd volunteered to search for a venue for the next WARP meeting. I'd just been really busy. But things at work were going to ease up within the next couple of days, I explained to Linda, who was a board member as well as the newsletter editor. "I'll get to it then," I assured her.

"We'd be happy to help." She sounded concerned.

There was no reason for her to worry. In fact, I was quite miffed. *Why doesn't she trust me to do the job? Does she think I'm incompetent?*

"No, no, I'm fine. I'll get to it next week."

"Are you sure?"

"Oh, absolutely. No worries. I'll definitely get to it." And I truly meant it; I knew that I would get to it.

But I didn't get to it the following week, or the week after, or the week after that.

My problems with initiating tasks go far beyond procrastination. The end result is essentially the same, but task-initiation glitches and plain old procrastination feel completely different.

Before the surgeries, after I'd completed a big project, such as a grant proposal or weaving yardage, I often had trouble finding the impetus to start on a new task. Even if it was something relatively straightforward, like preparing for class or knitting a few rows on a sock, I'd have to work myself up to switching gears to get started. If the new project was more complex, it sometimes took me several days or even a couple of weeks before I managed to push myself to work on it.

Brain injury-related trouble with task initiation is a more extreme version. Instead of having to find the impetus, it's as if it was never there and must now be generated out of nothing. Switching gears to initiate a new task can take much longer than a few days, and the projects in question can all be minor, such as folding laundry after reading a page-turner, or starting a new chapter in a page-turner after folding laundry.

It's not a matter of not being in the mood for a particular activity, nor is depression the problem. I am neither lazy nor lethargic. In fact, when I am well rested, I am raring to go.

But even when I am wide-awake and fully functional, ready and willing to begin work on a new task, I may find myself incapable of doing so. I want to act but cannot, even if I have completed all the steps leading up to this new task and have prepared myself mentally. I fully intend to, I know I will, but I don't, I can't. It is as if a hex has been laid on me.

Launching into a new activity is the problem—nothing more, nothing less. Once I've initiated the task, I take off with it.

I cannot always anticipate when I'll have trouble or how long it will impact a particular task. I can be happily knitting a sock but, upon completion, be unable to start the second sock; then, out of the blue, several weeks later, I'll start the second sock. When knitting another pair, I may have no trouble whatsoever.

My neuropsychologist suggested that I write a daily list of problematic tasks and block off a chunk of time in my daily planner for each one. Because of my brain injury, I've also acquired a degree of rigidity, an obsessive-compulsive bent, which ensures that once I add a task to my list, I have to attend to it. Initiating the algorithm is the key that unlocks the door, and the rigidity is the force that propels me through it.

Unfortunately, I often have trouble identifying problematic tasks, because, in my mind, there is no problem; it is a fact that I will get to it, but not right now. I do not *think* that I will get to it, nor am I *convinced* I will; I *know* that I will . . . in a bit. Until my brain makes the connection that enables me to realize that this is a task I'm having difficulties initiating, there is nothing I can do consciously to remedy the situation.

More than a month after Linda offered to help me, I finally realized that the work I'd promised to do just wasn't going to happen. I could not bring myself to start the search for a venue for the WARP annual meeting. As soon as the awareness sank in, a wave of relief washed through me.

I phoned Linda. "You were right. I do need help; I can't bring myself to get to it."

Sometimes it takes me days before I am capable of acknowledging that I cannot initiate a particular activity, sometimes weeks or months. For all I know, there are such tasks that I have yet to add to the list.

Because of the self-defeating nature of the issue, identifying problematic tasks does not necessarily guarantee a cure, either. Occasionally, I've identified such tasks yet do nothing about them. I do not mark them down on my list or allocate times to take care of them, not because I don't want to, but because I can't—I can't initiate the algorithm to correct the problem.

I have yet to contact a cousin of mine with whom I used to exchange e-mails regularly, but since the surgeries, I have been unable to respond to any of his messages. We were close, and I honestly want to respond, but I just can't bring myself to do so. I will—I know that I will. Later, maybe tomorrow, maybe next year.

If only I could add e-mailing my cousin to the list . . . I will. Soon.

⌐

When I reach the top of the stairs, I hesitate for a split second. My cell phone continues to ring from downstairs. Expecting an important phone call, I throw all caution to the wind and rush back down.

Since my brain injury, whenever I stand at the top of a staircase, I pause, picturing myself falling, tumbling down head over heels, landing broken at the bottom. I see myself sprawled motionless at the foot of the stairs. At that point, I mentally shake myself and proceed downstairs cautiously, my hand on the railing, one careful step at a time.

But as the phone rings insistently, I'm too flustered to be as careful as usual, though I do keep my hand on the railing. I do not rush, as I would have prior to the brain hemorrhages—I do not run down; I do not skip steps—but today I walk down fluidly, quickly.

When I am halfway there, I know that I am moving too fast, that I won't be able to correct any unanticipated misstep.

I'm no longer good at transitions: waking up is a long, groggy process, adjusting to jet lag takes a month or so, rather than a few days, and I don't handle surprises well. I'm no good at transitioning from a fast, fluid motion to a complete stop. My brain is slow to send out signals, and the signals are slow to make their way to their destinations.

The phone stops ringing right when I land on the next-to-last step. As my brain tries to adjust to the silence, my balance becomes beyond precarious—I have insufficient control to take the next step safely. I know that I'm going to fall, but I don't have enough time to send the signals to minimize potential damage, to protect my head.

I stumble over the last step, and as my foot makes contact with the Moroccan rug at the bottom of the stairs, the rug slips out from under me and sends me flying. Terror grips me. I watch myself fall, and all I can do is hope that I won't hit my head hard.

Daniel, who has been sitting in the living room playing a game on his laptop, oblivious to his surroundings, hears the *whomp* as I land and leaps to his feet. "Mum! Are you okay? Did you hit your head?"

I'm lying in a heap on the floor, the rug crumpled under me, my cheek resting on the hardwood floor.

I am afraid to move, afraid to assess the damage.

But . . . I did not hit my head! I take inventory. Nothing really hurts.

I raise my head and grin. "I didn't hit my head! I'm okay! I'm fine!"

I hear Daniel's sigh of relief as I move to get up. "You mustn't run down the stairs! You really scared me. That rug has got to go! Now!"

Then he comes over and hugs me tightly.

⌒

I slowed down and wiped my face with my bandanna, as if I were wiping off sweat, in a surreptitious attempt to erase the evidence of my tears.

Joyce handed me back my paddle. "You should tell him."

I glanced at her. "Tell him what?"

Her gaze was fixed on Daniel, striding ahead of us. "He'll know something's wrong. You can't keep telling him you're fine whenever he asks, and he *will* ask."

"I don't want him to worry."

"He wants to help. You need to give him a chance to help. He deserves it."

But he was a kid, my kid; I didn't want to burden him. I didn't want to worry or scare him. It was my job to protect him, not his job to protect me.

My brain injury taught me to ask for help from many people, but not from my kids. I was still trying to hide as much as possible from them.

I often saw Daniel in the background, not hovering over me, not too close, but well within range. In potentially problematic situations, I occasionally felt the sweep of his radar. Whenever the bloody brain acted up and he was around, Daniel was immediately there, by my elbow, at the ready. But he always faded into the background if anyone else reached out to me.

I saw all this, but it never stuck long enough for me to make any connections. Until now, when Joyce reprimanded me.

She was right. In fact, both Daniel and Sarah were old enough to be of help. Daniel, at sixteen, often had the maturity and insight to ease my way quite effectively. Given that he witnessed more of my difficulties than anyone else, in many cases, he would probably be more helpful than most.

Joyce's nudge made me realize that by looking elsewhere for help, I was doing both kids a disservice. I was sending them the message that I did not trust them. And by shutting them out, I was being disrespectful.

Joyce, Daniel, and I had been on our way to dragon boat practice. I'd been locking the door when I'd realized the significance of today's date, August 9, 2008: my first surgery had been on August 8, 2007, and the second on August 10, 2007. With that realization came a wave of despair.

We headed over to the yacht club parking lot, our team's rallying point. Within minutes, Daniel was half a block ahead of us, his life jacket hanging off his shoulder and his paddle in his hand. He strode along in his own world while Joyce and I followed at a more leisurely pace.

Often, Joyce and I chatted the entire way, about the coaches, the previous practice, Daniel, our families, life. Other times, we strolled along in companionable silence, every so often breaking it with the odd remark about a rabbit, a bird, the height of the water in the creek, the weather.

This time, I was completely silent, unresponsive to Joyce's occasional utterances. I was fighting for control. I could feel my eyes become moist. I knew that once the first tear made its way up and over, there would be no stopping the flood.

I lost the battle approximately halfway to our destination.

"What's wrong?"

Incapable of speech, I just shook my head.

Wordlessly, Joyce pried my paddle out of my hand, placed both our paddles on the ground beside her, and drew me into an embrace. She held me until the sobs became hiccups and finally subsided altogether.

When I was ready to talk, I sighed. "I was between the two surgeries this time last year."

"You know that you're doing really well?"

"I know, but . . ."

"I know it's hard, but it's getting a lot better. Just look at you. You're back to dragon boating, you're a good paddler, you're strong."

I knew I was doing well, but there was still so much that was very wrong. I still woke up most mornings with vertigo. I still overloaded very easily. Shutdowns were frequent. And the unrelenting exhaustion . . .

I bent over to pick up my paddle. "We'd better catch up with Daniel; he'll start wondering."

By the time we rounded the corner and saw Daniel, the evidence of my distress should not have been apparent to those who didn't know me well. Daniel knew me well.

As we approached, Daniel peered closely at me. "Is everything all right?"

DEB BRANDON

My instinct was to smile and say that I was fine. "Not really."

"What's wrong?"

"It's my anniversary, the first year anniversary of my surgeries." My eyes brimmed over. "I'm a bit of a mess over it."

"Do you need a hug?"

I nodded.

As Daniel moved to envelop me in his arms, the dam broke again. My tears flowed steadily, silently. He kept his arms around me until I shifted my weight away from him.

"You ready?"

I squared my shoulders. "Uh-huh."

Side by side, Daniel towering over me, his arm around my shoulders, we strolled toward the throng of our fellow teammates.

A cluster of breast cancer survivors congregated between us and the rest of the team.

Our dragon boat team, the Steel City Dragons, includes a team of breast cancer survivors, named Pink Steel. Breast cancer survivor teams are very much a part of the dragon boat scene. The repetitive paddling motion is effective in both reducing scarring in and rebuilding muscles affected by lumpectomies or mastectomies. As an added bonus, these teams provide a forum that enhances mental and emotional recovery.

Although I did not paddle with Pink Steel, they offered me much needed support when I returned to dragon boating after the surgeries. The emotional aspects of our paths as survivors were very similar, and they understood my journey in ways many people could not.

Julie, a Pink Steel member, was unloading her car. Her brief greeting set the tears rolling down my cheeks again. Ruth and Gay, also breast cancer survivors, converged on me. "What's going on?"

"It's my first anniversary."

Gay hugged me. "The first is the hardest. It hits you in the face."

Ruth nodded. "I guess it's part of what we have to go through to accept it."

Gay added, "Trying to see it as a celebration of how far you've come helps. And look how far you've come. Think back to the early days."

"I didn't really notice the second anniversary. A few days later, I realized it had come and gone." Ruth chuckled.

I'd lost track of Daniel while talking to Ruth and Gay, but when I turned from them to continue on my way toward the docks, he was right there by my side.

The heat slammed into me as I stepped out of the dragon boat.

I've never done well in hot weather, even during the days before my life turned upside down. Since the surgeries, I've become much more susceptible to neurological side effects. I do not consume alcohol; I avoid bug spray; I wear a hat when I am out in the sun.

During this summer, three years postsurgery, I had discovered that I'd become prone to heat exhaustion.

We'd had several long stretches of hot, humid weather, longer than is usual for our region. I'd suffered from heat exhaustion a couple of times and had to absent myself from several dragon boat practice sessions.

Now, we were in Cleveland, racing on the Cuyahoga River. The temperature was in the hundreds, and the humidity was so high that I had trouble sucking the air into my lungs. I was awaiting my turn to climb out of the boat after the race, the sweat dripping off my face, trickling between my skin and clothing, pooling in the creases, leaving wet patches on my shorts and T-shirt.

Patty, my seatmate, handed me her paddle and clambered out, gripping the hand of the volunteer who'd been helping with the docking. Once she stood safely on the dock, he let go of her hand and turned to me. I handed Patty her paddle and added mine to it. I slid along the seat toward the gunwale closest to the dock and gripped it hard in one hand, readying myself. The volunteer offered me his hand.

In the dragon boat world, someone always offers a helping hand at the end of a practice or a race. Some paddlers accept the help, and others decline. In the past, before the hemorrhages, I'd always declined the offers.

Now, I accepted the volunteer's proffered hand readily, automatically.

Our hands were twined around each other as I gripped his wrist and he gripped mine. He gave a little tug, and I followed his lead as he guided my momentum. As soon as my weight started shifting away from the boat, he gave me access to his shoulder in case I needed additional support. I leaned on it heavily as I shifted my weight and mentally rehearsed the steps needed to gain my equilibrium on the floating docks. They swayed with every motion of the choppy waters, so it would take me a few seconds longer than usual to steady myself.

As I stepped onto the docks, the effect of the heat smashed into me full force. My mental preparation was worthless. I had no balance to speak of. Despite his shoulder, I started to topple. He caught me.

This was the first time a complete stranger had come to my rescue. I'd known that at some point I would find myself in such a situation. I'd been dreading it; I couldn't bear the thought of going through a long, convoluted explanation, only to see discomfort or pity in a stranger's eyes.

I smiled my thanks. "I have balance issues."

No more explanations were needed. He stood up, his arm supporting me. He walked with me along the dock, holding on to me until we reached firm ground, the steps up to the boardwalk, then asked, "Are you okay from here on?"

My hand firmly gripping the rail, I grinned, tested my balance, shifting from one foot to the other, and nodded.

I was definitely okay, in more ways than one.

chapter twenty-two

2008–2009:
Scars

MOTIVATED BY MY AVERSION TO THE CROP-CIRCLE look, I decided to shave my head bald prior to the surgeries.

Sarah practically had a meltdown when I told her. "You'll look like a freak," she wailed.

"They'll shave it in the hospital anyway, but only patches, which would look really freaky."

But Sarah was adamant. "Promise me you won't shave it all off."

She had enough on her plate—she understood the risks involved in the surgeries—and I didn't want to add to her distress. We compromised. Instead of shaving it, I'd get a really close buzz cut. I was actually somewhat relieved by the change in plan.

I knew I looked good with short hair. In the past, I had occasionally let it grow long, with the specific purpose of relishing the dramatic transformation when it was eventually cut short. But I'd never done anything as drastic as getting a buzz cut.

The first day I walked into Gaye's hair salon with my cane and explained to her about the brain bleeds, she told me about her son, Carson. He suffers from chronic hydrocephalus, commonly called water on the brain, and has undergone fifteen brain surgeries to drain the excess fluid. Consequently, I was more comfortable talking with her about my neurological issues than I was with anyone else. She truly understood my difficulties, and she always knew what to say and what not to say.

I kept my hair short after my first EEG. Since my hair grows quickly, I went in for a trim every three to four weeks. As a result, Gaye had monthly updates about my health and knew when my plans for the surgeries were finalized.

A couple of days before I flew to Arizona for the brain surgeries, I asked Gaye to buzz my hair.

She picked up her clippers, all business. "Carson always asks me to shave his head before surgery."

She buzzed my hair down to less than a quarter of an inch yet still managed to give it style, emphasizing my widow's peak. I loved it.

She wouldn't accept money, and before I left, she gave me a hug and said, "Come back safe."

A few weeks after I returned from Arizona, I was back in the chair at the salon. Gaye was delighted that my hair had grown in so quickly. "You can barely see the scars. And that's only if you know where to look."

She addressed my reflection in the mirror. "So, what do you want me to do this time?"

"How about a buzz cut?"

Gaye shook her head vehemently. "Absolutely not! I'll cut it short, but I won't buzz it."

I felt as if I'd touched on a raw nerve; I assumed it was associated with the scars. Whether she refused because she did not want to be reminded of Carson's ordeal or because she was concerned that people would gawk at or be horrified by my scars, it didn't occur to me to question her.

A few weeks later, with my hair fluffing over my ears again, I was back in the hair salon. Gaye asked her usual question about what I wanted done. I grinned. "How about a buzz cut?"

She smiled and again politely refused.

For almost three years, every time I went in, I asked her for a buzz cut, and every time, she refused.

Finally, one day, Gaye wasn't in. Her daughter, Shelly, also a hairdresser, stood in for her. Here was my chance!

Shelly asked, "What would you like to have done?"

I grinned. "How about a buzz cut?"

She laughed. "Mom warned me you'd ask, and she told me not to do it. She made me promise."

I let out a deep sigh of resignation.

I was shocked and ashamed by the wave of envy that struck me when Betty said, "Photo Lynn wants to take pictures of my scars. I don't know if I feel comfortable doing that."

I stammered an acceptable response. "I-I'm not sure how I'd feel in your place, either."

Betty, my next-door neighbor and fellow dragon boater, was standing at the foot of the steps to my front porch. She'd caught me just as I reached my door.

She added, "She's doing some sort of project about scars. She's already taken photos of a couple of other Pink Steel women."

Another wave hit hard, a larger one. I imagined Betty standing in front of a mirror, lifting her shirt to study the aftermath of her mastectomy. I didn't care about the photos, the photographer, or her project—this was about the scars.

Photo Lynn, as the women of Pink Steel called her, so as

not to confuse her with Coach Lynne, was a photojournalist. A freelancer for *Sports Illustrated*, she'd spent the dragon boat season following Pink Steel's practices and races, photographing the team on and off the water.

She'd asked Betty and a couple of other Pink Steel women who hadn't had reconstructive surgery whether they'd be willing to let her photograph their scars. And I envied them.

Unlike the women on the breast cancer survivor team, I could not see my scars clearly in the mirror. I could not examine them closely. I could not poke and prod them while I watched them pucker and stretch. I had no way of imagining them, their color, shape, or length. Was there a sheen to them?

My hand often strayed up toward my right ear, my index finger drawn to the exposed tail end of the scar from the brain stem surgery, the scar that extends downward from behind my ear to an inch below my hairline. I'd absentmindedly trace the scar with my fingertip, starting with the narrow ridge of the tail that lay along the bottom of a channel-like indentation, then run upward over a couple of bumps, feeling my way through a forest of hair, and into a shallow basin above my ear. I'd rest my finger there, applying pressure, massaging; then I'd trace the line back down to the tip of the tail.

Once my finger recognized the starting point, the tail, I'd anticipate every twist and turn, every bump, every change in texture. I knew the scar well despite never having seen it with my own eyes.

What did those bumps my fingers knew so well look like?

Within a couple of hours of the first two brain surgeries, my brother Jonathan had snapped before-and-after photos. The images were grainy—he used his cell phone—though detailed enough to convey the gruesomeness of my wounds.

After my conversation with Betty, I searched for the images in my computer files.

I smiled at the first picture—a photo of a cactus wearing a hat and sunglasses, standing outside the hospital. Next was a photo of the X mark on my right temple, made to ensure that the surgeons wouldn't cut open the wrong side, which would have been bad, very bad.

I leaned in closer to the screen to study the after pictures. I pored over those grainy snapshots, scrutinizing the red, angry, blood-encrusted lines that crossed my scalp. I was puzzled, trying to understand—it was as if they belonged to someone else, a stranger.

My need to see my scars grew like a river collecting tributaries. I now wanted to see both scars, in their entirety. The idea of shaving my head was becoming attractive.

Judy suggested that I have someone photograph a panoramic view of my head that I could hang up on the wall and study at will, until I was satiated.

I imagined a series of black-and-white photos lined up side by side. I wondered about having daily photos of the scars as my hair grew in, mimicking the healing process.

Thinking about it reminded me of a book by a colleague of mine from Carnegie Mellon, Charlee Brodky, a professor in the school of design. In the book, *Knowing Stephanie*, Charlee told Stephanie's story of life with breast cancer through photographs. Some of the photos were of scenes when Stephanie had her head shaved in preparation for chemotherapy. I'd bought the book years earlier. I pulled it out and found the images more breathtaking than I remembered.

I wanted something breathtaking.

I wanted art.

But I was a weaver and a math professor, not a fine-art photographer. Was I completely off base? Did my idea have any artistic merit?

Seeking input, I turned to Photo Lynn. I showed her the book to give her an idea of what I had in mind.

Her eyes lit up. "That's a great idea! It could make for an interesting project."

I envisioned a string of pictures in different dimensions, hanging against a white background. I saw a series zooming in on one scar, then out, then in again on the other scar, and out again. I pictured black-and-white images beside their colored versions.

But who should photograph the scars? Joyce offered, but I wasn't sure of her prowess as a photographer. She'd certainly produced some great photos in the past, but I was skeptical about her ability to produce art. I thought of Photo Lynn, but I knew she was extremely busy, more often than not on the road. Charlee was a possibility.

Still tentative about shaving my head, not absolutely sure of my commitment to such a project, I postponed taking the first step.

After letting the idea simmer over the next couple of weeks, I was ready to ask Charlee whether she had any interest in such a project. I didn't have her phone number at home, so I planned to phone her from my office the next day.

That evening, I happened to see Photo Lynn, who greeted me by saying, "If you decide to shave your head, I'd be interested in photographing it."

I was thrilled by her offer, but I had some concerns I needed to address before I started figuring out the logistics.

The main obstacle was Sarah. I couldn't shave my head without warning her in advance. Dreading her reaction, I waited for the right moment but soon realized that there was no such thing. I finally just dove in.

She was reclining on her bed, working on her laptop. I poked my head in the door. "I'm planning on shaving my head."

She raised her eyes to stare at me. "Why?"

"I'm working on a joint project with a photographer who will be taking pictures of my scars."

Sarah arched her eyebrows. "Why would you want to do that?"

"I need to."

She turned back to her computer screen. "I'm not going to like it."

I chose to read into her reaction a grudging consent.

Seeking more positive input, I mentioned the project to my niece Ella, who was majoring in photography at the time. She responded with a delighted, "Oh, cool!"

Given that the fall semester was about to begin, I was concerned about reactions from incoming students, wondering whether I should try to squeeze the photo shoot in sooner, rather than later. I spoke to our undergraduate student advisor. He echoed Ella's enthusiasm.

My sister, Rachel, a long-time buzz-cut aficionado, was merely curious about my motivation, and Ferna, my secretary, just seemed puzzled.

A student who'd overheard my discussion with Ferna said, "That's awesome!"

At that point, all my hesitation vanished.

But who should shave my head?

I imagined photos of me during the shaving process, then photos focusing on the scars. So perhaps it should be split into two sessions: one in the salon, in front of a mirror, while I was being shaved; the other . . . in my house? On my porch? Or perhaps we could do it all in the hair salon?

I was sure that Gaye would say no. I thought of going to a barbershop, but somehow that seemed too impersonal.

Joyce offered to do the deed; she'd shaved a friend's head a couple of times. Did I trust her to do a decent job? Surely it wasn't possible to do an indecent job.

I wanted Joyce with me anyway. Because, in the wake of the brain injury, I had become much more emotionally volatile and vulnerable, the combination of my growing excitement over the project and residual twinges of trepidation about shaving my head were bound to get out of hand. The chances that overload would strike me during the shoot were extremely high. I trusted Joyce to help me through it. Also, if Joyce were to shave me, we'd be able to go through the entire process at home, in private, which felt right to me.

Joyce was as excited as I was. "How about after I shave you, I follow the lines of your scars with markers?"

I added, "Like a pirate, with little line segments crossing the big ones."

She laughed. "I assume you want washable markers; I think I have some at home."

I was primed and ready for this adventure.

It becomes harder to follow Lynn's instructions. "Turn your head that way, away from me." I move it slowly, in smaller and smaller increments.

"A bit more." I'm not sure I'll make it. Half an inch, another, a quarter . . .

"That's good."

I feel my facial muscles slacken as time slows down. I'm overloading, and Lynn can't see me through the camera. *Where's Joyce?* I'm not sure what to do. *What if Lynn wants me to move again? Where's Joyce?*

I hear the screen door squeak, then bang shut, and Joyce reappears. She looks at me sharply. "You okay?"

I plead with my eyes.

She closes the distance between us in a couple of strides. "We're losing her." The clicking of the camera hesitates for a split second, then resumes.

Joyce asks, "You want me to finish it off?" I blink slowly.

"Okay, I'll be quick as I can."

I wonder if the clippers are blunt—I feel the tug on each strand of hair as they do battle with it. My scalp fights to hold on to every strand. There is no relief—as soon as the clippers release one strip of hair, they capture the next, pulling and tugging. The inflamed follicles are setting my scalp on fire. I am all pain. I want to ask Joyce to stop, but I cannot.

"We're getting there. Almost done."

My eyes are brimming with tears. The clicking of the camera continues.

I can't bear another moment of this searing pain. My tears are about to overflow. And . . . my brain shuts down.

"We've lost her."

I hear a sharp intake of breath to my right, from Lynn's direction. The camera pauses for a long moment in its clicking.

In contrast, Joyce is all action—she catches my head before it droops all the way down to my chest and cradles it in her hand while propping my torso against hers, preventing me from collapsing onto the floor. I feel every ridge of the swirls of her fingertips on my cheek, every line on the palm of her hand. I feel the warmth of her skin sink into mine.

The clicking of the camera picks up again. I hear the split-second pause while Lynn presses down with her finger, I hear the shutter open and close; I hear the split-second hesitation as she releases the button.

Time slows almost to a stop. I lose track—one minute, two minutes, five, maybe even ten . . .

I spring back to life, popping out of the shutdown as my eyes open. The world around me resumes its flow. I smile an apology. Joyce tidies up, running the clippers once more over a couple of longer patches, snipping off stray strands with scissors.

She hands me a compact mirror. I grab it and hold it up. I tilt my head this way and that, moving the mirror up and down, side to side, trying different angles. "Where is it? I can't see it."

I have no interest in the brain stem scar. I'm searching for the bigger one, the one from the large angioma in the parietal lobe, the one I've never seen, have never been able to locate by touch.

Joyce points, but I can't see it in the tiny mirror. She guides my fingers. Lynn continues to take pictures as I hunt frantically with my fingertips. I feel a dent, larger and deeper than the one from the brain stem scar. I search in the mirror, but it isn't there.

I hear myself whine, "I want to see it. You'll need to cut more off. You need to shave it; you have to."

The clicking stops. Lynn rises from her crouch and holds out her camera. "Here, look at this photo."

I study the small LCD screen, but I don't understand. She points to a Y-shaped shadow, the shadow of the scar I'm so desperate to claim as my own. I feel a jolt, and something shifts inside me. I let out the breath I've been holding and break into a grin. "That's it! That's what I needed to see."

Like a dog circling on a bed searching for the right spot, finally finding it and settling down for a nap with a sigh of contentment, I feel a calm settle over me. I realize there's been a restlessness inside me for a very long time.

Joyce bundles up the sheet we've used as a hairdresser's gown and carries it outside to shake the hair out. I climb the stairs to the bathroom to study my reflection in the mirror on the medicine cabinet.

My entire face is framed in the large bathroom mirror. I stand in front of it, mesmerized, stroking my head, delighting in the silkiness as I run my hand in the direction of growth, the hedgehog prickliness as I go in the opposite direction. Almost of its own volition, my hand brushes back and forth, back and forth, as I gaze at my image, a goofy expression on my face.

As Lynn joins me, camera at the ready, I tilt my head, trying to see the Y-shaped scar in the mirror. Unable to see it, I open the cabinet doors.

I experiment, angling the mirror-lined doors in different ways, turning my head this way and that, while shifting my gaze from one reflection to the next in the various mirrors. After a long moment, I locate the shadow of my Y-shaped scar. I can see it, with my own eyes.

I close my eyes and feel for it with my fingers. There's the indentation. I open my eyes, smile at my reflection, my fingers still on the scar, and let out a deep sigh.

I go back downstairs, expecting to sit back down for the second phase of the operation: shaving my head clean. But Joyce has cleared everything away—the sheet, the stepstool I was sitting on, the clippers—and she's swept up all the hair.

Lynn, too, seems to be wrapping up. I'm a bit puzzled but shrug it off. Shaving my head completely is no longer important—I've found what I needed. It's there. I can see it. I have validation. It's mine, a part of me.

When my photo shoot was over, Lynn had to hurry to the yacht club to meet with Pink Steel. Having trouble finding enough words to express my gratitude, I hugged her fiercely before she took off. When I reentered the house, a beaming Joyce greeted me. I responded with a broad grin of my own, and a giddiness took hold of me. I couldn't stay still; I wanted to dance, to skip, to celebrate.

I wanted to share this landmark with people who would require little explanation, who would know that this was a celebration of life. I thought of the women of Pink Steel. My only hesitation was that, as breast cancer survivors, they might associate my buzz cut with cancer. But they knew me; they'd understand the real story.

Pink Steel members were milling around in the yacht club parking lot, waiting for Coach Lynne before they headed off for the boats. When they caught sight of Joyce and me, they swarmed us, welcoming smiles on their faces. Ruth ran her hand over my scalp. "Why the buzz cut?"

"I needed to see my scars."

Several of them nodded and laughed in congratulation. Darlene, a few inches shorter than I, peered up at my head as if she were nearsighted. "Where are the scars?"

I turned my head, and Joyce pointed them out. Out of the corner of my eye, I caught sight of Photo Lynn snapping away with her camera.

Coach Lynne sauntered over. "What's the deal with your hair?"

I told her how Pink Steel had helped me through my emotional recovery from the brain injury, how they'd been there for me during my first anniversary. I explained about the photo shoot and that I had wanted to share my experience with them.

She smiled. "And it's on your third anniversary as well. That's pretty cool."

My third anniversary. I'd completely forgotten. The timing *was* pretty cool, especially since the two events had coincided simply by chance.

A few weeks later, Photo Lynn stopped by to hand me the CD with all the photos. "You should have someone with you when you look at these. Someone you trust."

I looked at her askance, but she did not elaborate.

I was mystified but willing to take her word for it.

Of everyone I knew, Cindy and Joyce were the only ones I trusted implicitly. Cindy was in Colorado, and Joyce was leaving for Israel in a few days and had company until then. Could I wait the two months until Joyce returned from her trip? Did I really need to wait? Why had Lynn warned me not to view the photos on my own? Was she being unnecessarily cautious, even melodramatic?

After Lynn left, the CD and I stared at each other. I turned my back on it and went upstairs, leaving it on the coffee table in the living room. It called me. I tried to ignore it, but it was insistent. I went back downstairs, picked it up, put it back down, then picked it up again and held it. Wait a couple of months to look at the photos? I carried it upstairs.

I placed the CD and my phone by my laptop, which sits on my desk, no more than a yard from my bed. I set conditions before I allowed myself to pop the disc into the laptop: I was to keep tabs on my psyche throughout, and at the first sign of trouble, I was to phone Joyce to help me through any emotional distress, and I was to make my way over to the bed in case I shut down.

I slid the CD into the laptop and clicked to view the images. I took a deep breath, released the tension in my neck and shoulders, and started going through them one by one, slowly, methodically.

As I pored over the pictures, I was filled with wonder at how much I could read into them, how each photo clearly revealed my emotions and my state of mind.

Most images were headshots of me with varying amounts of hair: a full head, partially buzzed, practically bald. In some, I was trying to capture my scars in the small mirror or searching for them with my fingers. Joyce appeared in many, shearing, pointing, guiding.

In a couple, I looked old and weary. When I studied them carefully, I noticed my slackened facial muscles, which, according to Joyce, were one of the outward signs that I was overloading and about to shut down.

I froze and forgot to breathe as I stared at myself in full shutdown: the image of me slumped over, my head cradled in Joyce's hand. I looked so still, comatose, as if my essence had been extinguished. But I was in there, very much alive—my sense of hearing and my sense of touch were highly attuned to my surroundings, more so than usual.

This empty husk was what outsiders saw when I was in a shutdown. No wonder people freaked out.

I finally exhaled, hesitated for a couple of seconds, and moved on to the next photo and the next, a series of images of me in shutdown. As I clicked through the series, the initial impact of seeing that empty husk eased. I searched for a photo of me popping out of the shutdown but couldn't find one. I shrugged it off—Lynn must have missed that moment, or I just didn't recognize it in photos.

In the vast majority of the pictures, my face was expressive. In image after image, I was curious, intrigued, frustrated, desperate, relieved, happy, giddy—I was full of life.

Every few images, I paused to take inventory. *Are there any signs of tears? Am I swallowing hard when confronted by any of the photos? Is my breathing even? What about my heart rate?*

At several points, the answer to a couple of those questions was yes. Each time, I paused, leaned back in my seat, took a deep breath. As soon as I determined that all potential signs of difficulty had faded, forgetting my promise to lie down at the first sign of trouble, I pushed on.

I surfaced from examining all 308 of those pictures as if in a trance, staring blankly at the screen. My mind was a void, and the images were gone. I knew they were locked in one of my internal file cabinets, but I had absolutely no access to them. The only remaining trace was the knowledge that they were there somewhere.

The world around me ground to a glacial pace. I sat very still, my breathing so shallow that my chest hardly moved.

I emerged from my stupor gradually, the world still sluggish, all my thoughts, emotions, and movements in slow motion.

Abruptly, my limbs and eyelids became unbearably heavy. It took an eternity before I identified the heaviness as a symptom of exhaustion, and another extended delay before I recognized that the sudden-onset fatigue was probably a warning of imminent shutdown. A lifetime later, I realized that I should lie down. It took eons to reach my bed.

I lay on my back, the covers pulled up to my chin, unmoving, staring but unseeing.

Was I asleep? I felt groggy, as if I were waking up. I looked at the clock; an hour had gone by. I must have fallen asleep. But it didn't feel like sleep; it felt more like an absence. It reminded me of general anesthesia. There was no transition between awareness and absence; it was as if someone had flipped a switch.

I looked at the clock again; two more hours had passed. I must have just emerged from another absence. Although I now felt as if I belonged in the present, I stayed in bed a few minutes longer in case I had another relapse. Once convinced I was okay, I got up.

I spent the following couple of hours writing, then, drowsy in the normal sense, I went to bed and fell asleep, regular sleep. When I woke up in the morning, I felt an overwhelming urge to cry.

After my sobs faded away, I tried to recall the previous afternoon's photo-viewing session. I found no more than wisps of memories.

I recalled a few facts. I remembered that tears had come close to the surface over a couple of the photos. I remembered having studied my expression in each photo and that I'd been filled with a sense of wonder at how much emotion I could read into them. I remembered having marveled at Lynn's ability to capture my expressions so vividly.

But I could not remember the photos themselves; it was as if they had never existed. I could not recall a single one of them, not even a hazy impression.

I was afraid. My reaction had been too extreme. I put the disc away. I wasn't ready to view them again to fill the void, not on my own. I would wait until I had someone beside me. Someone I trusted.

Months went by before I remembered that disc. By then, I'd forgotten how severely I'd overloaded and shut down. I'd lost my apprehension and fear. I decided to have another look.

I sat down at my computer and, without any preamble—no deep breath, no releasing tension in my neck and shoulders, no one and no phone beside me—clicked the file open. I ran through the slideshow twice and felt . . . lost.

I searched to find myself in those images. I felt detached from them. I had trouble identifying the cascade of emotions I had experienced when the camera had been clicking away. The only memories they evoked were factual—they were sharp, beautifully detailed, but merely photos.

Now, a couple of years since the photo shoot, I view the slideshow once more. I examine my expressions in the images, identifying the emotions associated with them, recognizing the changes in my state of mind. But I also study Joyce—her stance, her expressions, her hands. I chuckle at the tabby cats in red high-tops marching across the sheet that covers me from the neck down. I notice the backgrounds. I study the various angles, the poses, the composition, the artistry. I smile at some photos, sigh at others, fly past many of them, and linger over a few.

Unbidden, my forefinger traces the line of the scar from my brain stem surgery. I have found myself in those images once again.

chapter twenty-three

2008–2009:
Filters

I WANTED TO SCREAM; I WANTED TO PUNCH SOMETHING; I wanted to throw things.

I could feel the rage building up inside me, a roiling, black, thunderous cloud, surging, threatening to escape. I knew that if I didn't keep it contained, I would lose all control. I would become the storm, destroying everything in its wake.

The paddler who sat in front of me at dragon boat practice had annoyed me. As I stewed over it on my way home, the irritation escalated, and by the time I walked in the door, I was seething.

Joyce and Sarah were sitting in the living room, waiting for me, looking at me expectantly, looking to me to . . . what? To take charge? To come up with a plan for the rest of the day? The rage exploded inside me. *What the hell are they waiting for? I'm tired. Why can't they leave me alone?*

I glared at them and noticed, through a chink in my fury, that Sarah's skin had a pasty look to it, and her eyes were dull. Oh, yes—she'd had a bad headache. She had come home from a sleepover with a horrific migraine.

I made a gargantuan effort to rein in the rage. "How's your head?"

I fought hard to listen to her response. I could hear the winds howling in my head, whipping the storm into a frenzy. I felt a scream pushing up my throat.

I had to do something. Perhaps I could fool the furor into dissipating by holding a seemingly reasonable conversation. I took a deep breath and turned to Joyce. "Guess where I sat in the boat?"

"You sat in the first seat?"

I shook my head, my teeth clenched.

"In the back?"

This was no rational dialogue: Joyce's responses were infuriating me. I couldn't play this game. The muscles in my jaw worked as I ground my teeth. "No. I paddled on the right. You know how I hate sitting on the right. I have neither power nor endurance when I sit right. And the person in front of me was pushing the rate. I can't stand it when people push rate. It messes up the whole boat. Why can't they follow first seat? She was in second seat. Her job is to prevent the rest of the boat from pushing the rate."

"I know what it's like. I often come away frustrated when people don't follow—"

"Lynne and Peggy were sitting first seat." My voice rose. "When I tried to follow Lynne, the woman clacked paddles with me. I couldn't reach. I couldn't get a full stroke. I can't stand it when that happens."

I opened my mouth to continue, then closed it, frowning and shaking my head. It was pointless—the words brought no relief.

I wanted to shriek. I needed to shriek.

I breathed in deeply, and as I let the air out, I tried to imagine the muscles in my neck and shoulders melting.

Sarah chose that unfortunate moment to ask, "When can we pick up Julia?"

Lightning struck; I balled my hands into fists, gritted my teeth, and snapped, "After I take a shower."

"Can we get lunch afterward? I asked Joyce to join us?" Her voice was small but determined.

The air crackled with electricity. But through the black clouds there was a trace of sanity, a flicker of a memory: before practice, I had promised her that we would go.

I didn't have the energy to fight the urge to hurt her. I didn't want to lash out at either her or Joyce, and I knew that if I stayed downstairs, it was inevitable that something would trigger additional lightning.

I turned on my heel and stomped up the stairs.

Perhaps a shower will help. I don't care if Sarah becomes impatient. I'm sweaty and stinky and furious.

I took my time. My actions were slow and deliberate: adjusting the temperature carefully; choosing the shampoo; lathering, rinsing, and rinsing once more. I stood under the showerhead for a couple of minutes, my face tilted upward, my eyes closed, letting the water run down me, willing it to cleanse me of the fury.

It was to no avail. If anything, the water was churning up the muck in the recesses of my mind, bringing it to the surface, adding to the debris already tossed around by the tempest.

The battle to maintain control was draining my energy, threatening to deplete my already low reserves. It felt as if I were putting all my weight against a door, trying to prevent gale-force winds from wrenching it open. I was tiring; my grip on reason was loosening.

All my muscles were tight, tense with rage. I dried myself and dressed, every movement a strain, every motion jerky.

I wanted the torrential rains to abate, the thunder and lightning to cease. I wanted to calm down. I wanted to rejoin Sarah and Joyce as a human being, not as a raging storm.

I knew that I shouldn't go directly downstairs. I had to stall for time; I had to find a way to quell my fury.

I sat at the computer. *Perhaps if I write* . . . Writing always soothes me when my emotions run high.

I started: "I wanted to scream, I wanted to punch something, I wanted to throw . . ." when Sarah called, "Are you ready to go?"

Immediately, my shoulders tensed up and my jaw muscles tightened. *I want to write! I need to write! Instead, I'm expected to cater to everyone else. That is it!* I barked, "Yes, I'm coming!"

I snatched up my purse, grabbed the laundry basket, and stomped back downstairs.

Joyce asked me, "Do you know where we're going?"

I took a deep breath. "No, but we can take the GPS."

"Then we'd better take your car. My cigarette-lighter plug is a bit iffy."

I couldn't believe my ears. *She knows I don't like driving, especially if I don't know my way. She knows I'm tired.*

Sarah again chose the wrong moment to open her mouth. "Can you give me the car keys?"

I gritted my teeth and dropped the basket onto the floor so that it would make a satisfying *thunk*. Yet I was not satisfied; nothing could satisfy me now. Another bolt of lightning struck, and another. I reached into my pocket, scrabbled for my keys, drew them out, and threw them at her forcefully.

And . . . she caught them, discharging another cluster of lightning bolts.

I stormed downstairs to the laundry room.

I flung the basket down on the floor by the washing machine, then raised my head to discover dry clothes strewn all over the machine.

"*Aaaarghhh!*" The scream erupted despite my attempts to

suppress it, and I almost broke into angry tears. I yelled, much more loudly than necessary, "Are these clothes on the washer clean or dirty?"

Joyce called out, "Clean!"

I'd known that she was the likely culprit. She had probably pulled the clothes out of the dryer when I'd asked her to bring me a clean towel earlier. But now that there was proof—an admission of guilt—she became the focus of my fury. *Why couldn't she just throw them back in the dryer after she found the towel? Why am I expected to do everything around here?*

I yanked open the dryer door, hurled the clean clothes in as hard as I could, and heaved the door closed with all the force I could muster. I pitched the clothes from the basket into the washing machine and turned it on, almost wrenching the knob off. I measured out the laundry detergent, spilling some, and dumped it in. I banged the lid down, turned, and strode stiffly through the garage and out toward the car, digging my nails into my palms, grinding my teeth, slamming every door that stood in my way.

I tore the car door open. Joyce and Sarah were already inside. I was so furious, I couldn't look Joyce in the eye. I threw myself into the driver's seat, banging my knees against the steering wheel, my eyes sliding away from Joyce's whenever we were in danger of making eye contact. I yanked the door closed and sat in the car in stony silence for a long moment, staring straight ahead.

As I jammed the key into the ignition, it occurred to me that perhaps I shouldn't drive in this state, but my fury squashed that thought flat almost as soon as it emerged. *I'll be fine! Anyway, Joyce made it clear that it would be better to take my car. So we're bloody going to take my car, and I'll be fine!*

As hard as I tried to keep the rage in check while I drove, I found myself hunched over the steering wheel, holding it in a death grip, my knuckles white, driving a bit too fast. I was jolted out of the worst of my fury when the car veered off the road briefly, but I was still caught up in the gale.

I had to regain control. *Maybe venting will help now.* . . .

I glanced at Joyce. "I tried to be patient with the woman in front of me, but I just couldn't take it anymore. I told her that she was pushing rate. She responded by saying that she was following Peggy. Can you believe it? Why do people feel the need to justify their ineptness? And so stupidly as well. She wasn't even supposed to be following Peggy; she was supposed to be following Lynne, like me. Anyway, if she was in fact following Peggy, then Peggy wasn't following stroke. Only after Lynne told her not to follow Peggy did she listen, but even then, when we really got going, she went too fast. What is wrong with people? Why do they let their rate run away with them? Why can't they maintain a semblance of control?"

The wind gusts let up somewhat. I could finally listen to Joyce, her words no longer triggering lightning, when she said, "You're preaching to the choir. I know how frustrating it can be."

The thunder was still rumbling. Another wrong surfaced. "During the kids' scrimmage, they were treating them like morons. Why do adults treat kids like morons? Don't they remember what it was like? Guess what? Kids are people, too, and they deserve the same level of respect as adults do. The coach was giving the adult team instructions on how to let the kids beat them. Not only was he not being subtle, but he was calling it out from the chase boat. Does he think they have cloth ears or something? They're not idiots. I hate it when grown-ups are like that around kids."

"I know what you mean."

My grip on the steering wheel loosened somewhat. The thunderclouds were lifting, looking much less ominous.

As the storm abated, fatigue set in. As with the other rages I have experienced since my brain injury, today's struggle to maintain my rationality had drained me dry.

I am not ashamed of becoming enraged; it's part of the brain injury package. Many brain injury survivors have issues with uncontrollable rage. Unlike the anger most people feel at times, these rages threaten to overwhelm us. Hanging on to our sanity requires major effort.

Anger and rage are related. Anger can act as a lead-in to rage, providing the trigger that sets it off. Often anger acts as a background while the rage bursts through it, sometimes once, other times more, sporadically, triggered again and again.

But they are completely different emotions. Anger never erupts without warning; it escalates, whereas rage explodes almost instantaneously, often unexpectedly and in full force.

Anger is never unmanageable; when I am angry, I am in full control the entire time, even when I'm slamming things around. But when I am enraged, I feel as if I am possessed by a demonic entity. I have to fight to ward it off, and often come alarmingly close to losing the battle.

Too many survivors are inadequately armed to withstand their rages, and when a storm strikes, it destroys everything in its path until the rage runs its course.

I am one of the lucky ones. I have become enraged no more than once every couple of months since my brain injury, and I have always eked out a victory in my fight to keep my fury in check.

The only memory I have of fully unleashing my rage is from long before the brain injury.

Throughout elementary school, I was noticeably shorter than my classmates, but it was of no consequence until Illana, in sixth grade, started referring to me as "adorable" or "cute." I found the affront to my dignity extremely annoying. The frequency at which she treated me so condescendingly grew, and with it, so did my irritation. But I said nothing.

However, when she pinched my cheek and said, "Oh, you're so cute!" I broke my silence. At first I asked her politely to stop, and she did . . . until the following day. When she did it a second time, I did not ask—I told her. That took care of it for a few days, but then she started pinching my cheeks again, giggling, "Oh, you're so adorable."

Finally, I snapped and yelled at her. But she just laughed.

The next day, she slapped me playfully, first on one cheek and then on the other. I froze. *No one slaps my face! How dare she! No one—no one—slaps me on the cheeks!* I held on to my temper, barely. My knuckles were white as my nails dug into my palms. Through clenched teeth, I told her to stop, but she just laughed. "Oh, you're so cute!" And she slapped me again.

All I could hear was roaring in my head. All I could see was lightning striking again and again.

There's a gap in my memory. The next thing I knew, she was kneeling prostrate on the floor, in the manner of a Muslim in prayer, while I jumped on her back. I remember that I felt confused and puzzled and horrified when I did regain my . . . what? My sanity? *What on earth am I doing? How did I get here? How did she get there?*

Luckily, she wasn't hurt. She never slapped me again. And I never completely lost control again.

The filters that I constructed over time to dampen raw emotions had been adjusted. The next time rage exploded, a finer mesh kept it contained.

I was fifteen years old. It was my turn to wash the dishes after dinner, and instead of getting to them right away, as I usually did, I procrastinated. When I finally came into the kitchen, Mum was standing at the sink, clacking dishes. I told her, "You can stop now. I'll do them."

She placed a plate on the rack and pulled another one out of the soapy water. "It's okay. I'm already doing them."

I gritted my teeth. "I'll do them." Then I heard myself add, "I want to do them."

She didn't turn around. "I've already started. I'll finish them."

I remember standing behind her, the roiling black skies in my mind lit by flashes of lightning. I balled my hands into fists. I envisioned picking her up and hurling her out of my way so that I could gain access to the sink.

That image stopped me in my tracks. *What the hell am I thinking?* And the tempest started dissipating. Not wanting to chance setting off additional lightning bolts, I turned my back on her and stormed off to my room.

That was the last time prior to my brain injury that I felt such overwhelming fury, when the battle to maintain control was so hard won. A heavier-duty filter had clicked into place.

More than thirty years later, the brain surgeries damaged those filters, and some days I revert to that enraged fifteen-year-old. I have to fight ferociously to contain my rage, but, like I did as a teenager, I always somehow manage to walk away without causing physical damage.

Rage is not a pretty emotion. Rage is objectionable, ugly, unpredictable, and sometimes dangerous. It's an unacceptable emotion: if we feel it, we are supposed to slam the lid down on it, immediately. It is socially inappropriate.

I am socially inappropriate. I always have been, to some extent, but I have become even more so since the brain injury.

I exhibit raw emotions, such as rage, and I have meltdowns, in public, among strangers. I swear more than many would consider appropriate. I generate conversations with strangers in elevators, I comment to fellow shoppers about their purchases, and I've been known to question passersby about their scars.

Sarah once mentioned to me that a friend of hers, Megan, was afraid that she was pregnant. The next time I saw Megan, she was working the cash register at a restaurant. As I was paying for my lunch, a line forming behind me, I questioned her about her use of contraceptives and whether she'd taken a pregnancy test. Only now, a couple of years later, as I write this, has it occurred to me that her workplace was not exactly the appropriate setting for such a discussion, and that perhaps our hushed conversation was not so hushed.

Had I been in a similar situation in the past, before the brain bleeds, I probably would have led a similar discussion, but I definitely would have known that it was not appropriate to hold it in public.

The effectiveness of the system of filters we construct over the years determines our behavior in a variety of situations. Input filters screen incoming data, such as social cues, and output filters regulate how we react. Our social input filters dictate how sensitive we are to incoming data, such as body language and tone of voice, and how aware we are of different cultural norms. Verbal output filters help us observe social niceties by regulating impulsive speech.

I could have taken at face value my mother's insistence on washing the dishes and remained completely oblivious to the subtler message she was projecting, and I would have gone to my room, happy that I'd escaped having to finish the chore. But my input filters were sophisticated enough for me to interpret her body language and tone of voice as the long-suffering-Jewish-mother act that it was, and I knew that she was trying to make me feel guilty. I reacted to that message with fury and stomped away. Instead, I could have confronted her more forcefully, possibly by swearing at her or with physical violence. Alternatively, I could have apologized for my procrastination, whether I meant it or not.

Filters do not act as separate entities; they work in conjunction with other filters. Sensory input filters interact to edit incoming information: what we see, hear, feel, smell, and taste. Emotional output filters regulate different emotions, which are also interconnected: anger and rage overlap, as do relief and joy.

The fineness of the mesh in the filters determines the effectiveness of the filtration process. Too fine a mesh in the emotional output filters may prevent us from expressing our emotions, closing us off from ourselves and the world. Too coarse a mesh releases every emotion like an uncontrolled flood. Too fine a mesh in our social input filters may block all social cues, making us oblivious to other people's emotions and reactions; too coarse, and we end up so sensitive that we read meaning when there is none and feel perpetually vulnerable or paranoid.

Presiding over the filters is our control center, guiding data through appropriate filters, directing messages from edited input toward output filters, and adjusting interactions between filters to achieve the optimal mesh size needed to accommodate a variety of situations. The more sophisticated the control center, the more flexible it is in handling unanticipated situations and the more quickly it responds to rapid changes in circumstances.

Throughout our lives, we build this complex system of filters that continually sifts through incoming and outgoing data, and we learn to improve our control center.

⌒

The bloody brain damaged my filtration system, undoing all the work I'd put into it since I was born. It seems as if the surgeries tore gaping holes in some of the meshes. Through these holes, strong emotions, impassioned speeches, or crude language pour out into the world. It also feels like the weave in some of the meshes is no longer uniform. I think of these meshes as a loosely woven fabric, like gauze, bulging out here, the weave more open there, and so tight in other areas that the holes are too small to let anything through.

With time, new filters have been constructed, completely re-placing some of the badly torn ones. But many of the filters have just been patched up. As with patching a hole in a pair of pants, if the hole is small, the patch can be almost invisible. When the hole is larger and jagged, the patch, though functional, will no-ticeably affect the flexibility and breathability of the fabric.

"Disinhibition"—a decrease in the ability to control impul-sive behavior—is a common consequence of brain injuries. Many brain injury survivors, including me, swear excessively.

The filters responsible for my verbal output were damaged, leading to increased profanity. During my first year postsurgery, I swore more than I ever used to, even more than I did as a teenager. An uncensored flow of expletives went hand in hand with frustrations and strong emotions, both positive and negative.

My control center was also affected. I was less careful around people, and all too often I tossed out swear words in casual con-versations, no matter how polite the company.

My impaired verbal output filters led not only to inordinate swearing but also to an extreme level of bluntness. I became much more outspoken and still often raise socially taboo subjects and verbalize uncomfortable truths.

I was speaking to Barbara, an employee of a funding agency that frequently provides financial support for the undergraduate research program I run every summer. I lamented the fact that many minority students are ill prepared for research in mathematics. I added that I refused to dumb down the program by admitting such students. I also told her that, unfortunately, some of these weaker students slip in through the cracks. But I also mentioned that, in our commitment to the success of all the participants, we address the issue by providing the weaker students with extra tutoring to bridge the gap.

Barbara is African American.

I believe that my reading of her social cues was correct, that that particular filter was working properly that day: her manner toward me did not change, she did not flinch or stiffen, and there was no change in her tone of voice. I felt no need to apologize. I'm sure that she did not take offense—shortly after I stepped down from my soapbox, she suggested that I apply for a sabbatical leave at her agency.

However, something was definitely wrong. As the words poured out of my mouth, I knew that I was committing a major political-correctness faux pas, but I couldn't stop myself. I knew I wasn't supposed to be so candid; none of my colleagues would have spoken so bluntly, especially to a person of color. Yet not only did I feel driven to continue, but I kept expanding and elaborating on the topic, repeating various points over and over.

I believe that prior to the surgeries, the input from Barbara's social cues, combined with my cultural awareness, would have produced a moderated version of my monologue. My argument would have been more linear, rational, and toned down.

I would have been much more careful with the wording, and I would not have been so repetitive.

My malfunctioning control center did not adjust mesh sizes appropriately: the mesh weaves were too fine in the cultural awareness filter and too coarse in the verbal output filter. In addition, although I was actually aware of the cultural inappropriateness, that information, that awareness, wasn't passed on to my verbal output filters.

Occasionally, my filtration control center, as with so many brain injury-related issues, behaves erratically. It is possible that the flood of words that soaked Barbara was due partly to one of the random blips in my control center. Out of the blue, either a wide gap will appear in a mesh, allowing a large chunk of data to pass through, or an arbitrary section in a filter will become blocked off, hampering the passage of signals.

The surgeries also badly affected the flexibility of my control center. It often takes longer to react than it used to, cutting down on the variety of situations it can handle and decreasing my ability to deal with surprises.

Imagine a situation where you are on the phone to a friend while your young kids are whining at you. You would not speak to your kids the same way you'd speak to your friend. Your tone of voice and the vocabulary you'd use would shift back and forth as you switched between speaking into the phone and handling the kids. The mesh in your cultural awareness filter would be in constant motion during your phone conversation, opening and closing. The meshes of your verbal output filters, corresponding to your tone of voice, your volume, the vocabulary you use, would also be opening and closing, depending on whom you're speaking to, your friend or your kids.

Since the surgeries, if I have to speak on the phone while dealing with another person by my side, my systems overload. I have difficulty switching back and forth between conversations and interacting with more than one person at a time.

My sensory input filters are particularly sensitive to overload. All too often, sometimes with no warning, they reach a point where they treat all input equally, without discrimination, inundating my neural pathways with a deluge of information that exceeds my brain's processing capacity. This large volume of unedited information clogs up my circuits, blocks off many of my filters, shorts out my control center, and causes total and utter mayhem.

In my case, "too much information" holds a less suggestive, more literal meaning than it does for most people.

Over the first few years postsurgery, my filters underwent some repairs and the frequency of my swearing decreased. Strong emotions still evoke swearing, but around those with more delicate sensibilities, I limit cursing to the occasional mild expletive. On the other hand, around people who are not uncomfortable with profanity, the swear words spew out of my mouth fast and furious, much more so than they ever did, as if behaving myself has been water rising behind a patched dam that's finally burst.

The repairs have been extensive, but most of the filters are not back to preinjury condition—a fact that I do not find distressing. Quite frankly, I would rather that these filters remain as they are now, even with their residual flaws. I am willing to live with my current level of emotional volatility and vulnerability, with the swearing and unvarnished honesty.

The fact that I refer to my filtration system as being damaged implies that the consequences are all negative. But that is far from the truth. For every negative, there is a positive.

Yes, the damaged emotional output filters allow rage to

erupt, but they also allow me fierce joy and deep compassion, an emotional intensity long muted. They bring a welcome brilliance into my life.

The impaired verbal output filters do cause excessive swearing and an outspokenness that can cause awkward situations. But my bluntness frequently acts as a much-needed icebreaker, opening lines of communication, making connections, possibly friendships, especially when it's combined with my newly intensified compassion.

If I were to complete the repairs on my filters, I'd suppress my outspokenness and tone down my heightened sensitivity to social nuances. I'd lose my ability to break down social barriers and my increased facility to read people, listen, empathize, and create deep bonds.

If profanity is the price for leaving those filters as they are, so be it. I'm quite happy to take the chance that some people will have trouble looking past the crude language to see me.

The damage to the sensory input filters also has benefits. While the dark chaos of sensory overload devours me, the temptation to repair the filters is there. But those damaged sensory input filters also let the world into my life in a rainbow of bright colors. They enable me to immerse myself in my surroundings and to absorb details I used to gloss over. I don't want to lose that hypersensitivity.

And how could I wish away my raw emotions? If my filters were fully restored so that I could better manage the rages, I might become shut off from the world again, from the vibrancy of life. I don't want to revert to viewing life through a fog of numbness.

The battles to control my rages are hard won, but I have managed to win every time. Some contained rage is acceptable, is it not?

chapter twenty-four

2010–2012:
You Win Some, You Lose Some

I SAT DOWN, OPEN BOOK IN HAND, AND STARED BLANKLY out the window. When my breathing was back to normal, I returned my gaze to the open page.

The print was small, the page dense with words. There was no way I'd be able to read it. I was in serious trouble.

I took a few deep breaths, squared my shoulders, and flipped through the book to the table of contents. I couldn't take it in; the words were meaningless. I rolled my shoulders, sat up straight, and took another deep breath. I ran over the list of contents, and a word jumped out at me: "determinants." I turned to that chapter, hoping that something familiar would catch my eye. A numerical example . . .

The fog in my brain lifted instantaneously: I knew how to find the determinant of a two-by-two matrix—my breathing quickened—and a three-by-three matrix. The tension in my neck and shoulders eased up a tad. I turned the page. The equation "det(AB) = det(A)det(B)" jumped into focus. I knew that. I relaxed. I could do this.

I closed the book with a snap and placed it in my shoulder bag. The book was coming home with me. I was going to work through it, exercise by exercise, chapter by chapter, day by day, until I was sure I'd be able to teach the material effectively. I'd done it before, during the first year after the surgeries; I'd do it again.

Stress didn't even begin to cover what I'd been feeling since I had found out about my teaching assignment for next semester, a course entitled Matrices and Linear Transformations. I'd taught a watered-down version of it in 2006, a year before the hemorrhages, but not since, and now, six years later, I was slated to teach a more abstract version—more theory, more proofs. Since the brain injury, I'd taught only the lowest-level math classes available at Carnegie Mellon University—first-year calculus courses for humanities and social sciences majors.

Finally, after a couple of years back in the classroom, I felt comfortable moving to higher-level courses, such as calculus for engineering and science students, but no higher, not yet. I certainly didn't feel ready for a course at the level of Matrices and Linear Transformations. I would have been anxious enough about teaching the earlier, easier version, which was already quite a leap in level from the humanities calculus.

John, our associate department head, makes all the decisions about the teaching assignments. Optimizing these assignments is no easy task. Every semester, he has to juggle teaching needs at the departmental and university levels, fitting instructors to the courses and the student population they are best suited for, while taking into account instructors' requests.

Teaching the calculus for humanities classes is not popular among my colleagues in the mathematical sciences department. A large percentage of humanities students have a history of struggling with math, many of them have issues with math anxiety, and most of them dislike the subject and see these required courses as a necessary evil. Having had an easy time learning calculus, many mathematicians have trouble empathizing with these students.

Before the brain bleeds, I enjoyed the students, but I did not particularly enjoy teaching them. I used to joke that it was calculus in slow motion. At the time, I was sure I was being as patient as could be, understanding and addressing their difficulties. I believed I did a good job. But now, having had to struggle to get back in the classroom, I am appalled at my past attitude and lack of empathy.

Now, I truly empathize with these students. I myself have panicked at a problem that required multiple steps; I, too, have stared at a clump of words and seen a tangle of knots that I couldn't unravel. I've had to learn to overcome that initial panic and solve the problem by finding a starting point and proceeding step by step.

I guide my humanities students through the steps I myself learned to follow. Given a word problem, I teach them to take a deep breath, start with the first sentence, and proceed line by line, translating the words into mathematical symbols and formulas. Next, I show them how to solve the problem, one step at a time.

By showing the students how to break problems into steps, I increase their awareness of the solution process and of the patterns that emerge. Thanks to my new need to find different approaches to problems, I'm better able to come up with explanations that make sense to students with a variety of thinking styles. At the same time, I am increasing their ability to approach any given problem in different ways. I am preparing them to solve a broader range of problems.

As I tell them at the beginning of each semester, I don't see familiarizing them with the material as the main goal of the course. My job is to help them hone their analytical thinking skills; learning calculus is merely a means to that end. I tell them that if they become adept at both linear and various types of nonlinear thinking, they will be able to grasp more of the bigger picture in their daily lives.

I have become passionate about teaching calculus for humanities and social sciences. I feel that I can make a real difference. I enjoy watching the students grow, not just academically but also personally, as the semester progresses. I love interacting with them; they are lively, interesting, and open-minded. They are much more socially adept than many other students, and once the semester is over, they do not treat me as if I am invisible. When we cross paths on campus, they make eye contact, acknowledge my existence with a smile, and usually stop to chat. Some of them continue to drop by my office to hang out and talk to me about their lives.

Despite my pronouncement that I felt at ease about upping the ante in my teaching assignments, John continued to assign me to teach the humanities classes for another year—he knew that no one else in the department fit that slot better than I did.

But now, I was a year away from renewal. When it's time to renew instructors' contracts, one of the items the faculty considers is the variety of courses an instructor teaches. Since the surgeries, I'd taught only the two lowest-level calculus courses. I needed to diversify my teaching assignments. Also, to counter possible concerns about my abilities in the wake of the brain injury, I needed to show that I was capable of tackling more advanced material.

John had been very accommodating since my surgeries, always working around my teaching preferences. He was ready to assign me to those humanities classes again, but this time I declined. I suggested that he have me teach one of the calculus courses for engineering and science majors. Instead, he assigned me to Matrices and Linear Transformations. And I was in a panic.

I spent several days working up the courage to approach him about my misgivings. Finally, I went to his office, expecting to discuss my concerns, hoping to work out an alternative, but he interrupted me midsentence, saying, "Anyone would be nervous teaching a new course like this."

John had never interrupted me like that before. He'd always listened to me patiently. Now, I got the distinct impression he didn't want to hear it. Perhaps his patience had run out. Did he believe that my reluctance to teach higher-level courses was now due to psychological reasons, rather than physiological ones?

I knew I'd been overly cautious in the past about upping the ante. But now, when it came to a course at this level, I wasn't so sure I was erring on the side of caution. I thought I was being realistic; at the very least, I lacked the confidence necessary for excelling in the classroom. I needed more time. I needed to build more slowly toward teaching such a course.

On the other hand, maybe John's abrupt manner wasn't about me. Perhaps he just needed to attend to some urgent business. Perhaps he was merely exhausted after a tough day, week, month. Or perhaps he felt that he'd finally sorted out the assignments and had his fill of dealing with instructors' requests and demands.

I knew that at this point in the game, assigning me to any of the calculus courses I'd requested would probably cause a major upheaval in the teaching assignments. John would have to rearrange the entire schedule and reassign several instructors.

I felt guilty about creating more work for John, but *my* issues were serious, were they not? My concerns weren't a matter of personal preference or convenience and surely should have taken priority over many other requests.

However, I didn't want to press the issue further. All the guilt I had about adding to his workload and stress levels and all the fears that had haunted me during my first year postsurgery came rushing back, engulfing me and my words. What if I wasn't ready? What if I wasn't up to it? What if I had to quit my job? Or, worse, what if I wouldn't be rehired?

During the next few months, whenever I was reminded of the upcoming semester, the fears surged through me like a tidal wave, filling every space in my being, leaving behind pools of anxiety.

I'd try to calm down, to think it through rationally, to break the cycle of fear. I was definitely okay with some of the material; certainly, that chapter on determinants would cause no difficulties, and I was fluent in Gaussian elimination. I tried to convince myself that the rest shouldn't be too hard. It was probably just a matter of recalling some of the topics from somewhere within the recesses of my mind.

I just had to work my way through the textbook, and I'd be fine.

I placed the textbook prominently on the dining room table, where I'd see it whenever I passed by.

Later that day, I walked through the dining room on my way to the kitchen and saw the book. I picked it up and opened it to the first chapter. The print was so small. . . . I'd look at it later.

I never opened it again.

Despite trying to convince myself that I could handle the material, deep down inside, I was still filled with self-doubt. My difficulties with the textbook itself merely added another layer to my distress. How could I possibly teach out of a book I could not read?

It occurred to me that I needed a large-print version of the book. But there was no large-print version. And large print alone wouldn't have solved the problem anyway—I'd learned that when my ability to read seemed not to have survived the surgeries.

I had always been a voracious reader. I could spend hours lost in a book, oblivious to my surroundings, fighting sleep as I read late into the night. I frequently became one with the characters in the story, sharing their lives, walking their paths.

I played croquet with the queen of hearts, as Alice in *Alice's Adventures in Wonderland*. I marched through the Malayan countryside, struggling to survive, as Jean in Nevil Shute's *A Town Like Alice*. While immersed in the *Harry Potter* books, I was Harry flying on my broomstick, my entire focus on the golden snitch. I bumbled along as Ron, and I sat in the library as Hermione, devouring books from cover to cover.

During my week in inpatient rehab, I progressed from understanding sentences to paragraphs to a one-page article—I was back to reading. And over the next few weeks, I finished the *Harry Potter* book I had brought with me to the hospital. I was back to being the avid reader I used to be.

Or so I believed.

Several months after I was discharged from the hospital, I noticed that my pile of unread books was not shrinking; in fact, it was growing. My book-buying habits had not changed since the brain hemorrhages, but my reading habits had.

Books that would have interested me in the past did not capture my attention. Unable to immerse myself like I had before, I only skimmed through them. I gravitated toward shorter books with more dialogue, less description, and minimal reflection—easy-reading books. Sometime in my second year postsurgery, I learned that brain injury survivors manage better with larger print. *Oh, so that's why I favor children's books!*

Cindy urged me to acquire an e-reader. "You could control the size of the print."

I scoffed at her advice. "It just wouldn't be the same as curling up in bed with a real book."

Soulless plastic is no substitute for wood; an electronic gadget could never take the place of a living book.

I couldn't conceive of flipping through a book without hearing the sound of paper rustling, without feeling the grain slide across my fingertips, dry and warm. I couldn't imagine reading without smelling traces of ink and dust awakened by air brushing across a newly opened page.

That summer, I became annoyed when Cindy repeated her suggestion. I told her, "I'd rather buy books in large print."

That was when, three years postsurgery, I finally made the connection: large print. The next time I visited a bookstore, I browsed through the large-print section and purchased a large-print version of a book I would have inhaled in the past.

That evening, almost ceremoniously, I brushed my teeth, washed my face, turned on my bedside lamp, switched off the overhead light, and climbed into bed with my book. I huddled under my blankets, turned to the first chapter, took a deep breath, and started reading.

I sighed as I completed the first page. *This is it!* With another sigh, I turned to the second page. But as I progressed through it, my enthusiasm flagged. It wasn't really holding my interest. *Maybe I'm too tired.*

I tried again the next day, but I just couldn't sink into the pages. I braved another book in large print, but to no avail: I was indifferent to it.

I surrendered and limited myself to easy-reading books. *It's not that great a loss. After all, there's no shortage of enjoyable easy-reading books.*

Except that it *was* a great loss, and I grieved every time one of those "other" books crossed my path.

It still didn't occur to me to consider an e-reader—I was too averse to the notion.

Ads for e-readers seemed to confront me wherever I went, yet I was not tempted. I always walked right past the e-reader display in the bookstore without giving it a second glance until I was in the store with a couple of bored teenagers: my daughter, Sarah, and her friend Jordon. They were idly investigating the e-readers while I hovered nearby. When an employee approached us, we fled, giggling.

Next time I went to the bookstore and passed the display, I picked up a pamphlet about e-readers. I'm not sure why. But when I got home, I promptly forgot about it.

On a subsequent trip, I glanced at the price list for the e-readers. *That's ridiculous! No one in her right mind would spend that kind of money on something like this!*

A few weeks later, I ambled into the bookstore with Daniel. An employee was discussing the e-readers with a customer. Curious, I lingered, eavesdropping. *It actually looks easy to use.* I contemplated the prices. *The cheaper one would suffice—I don't need all those other features.*

I asked, "How would you control the print size?"

The employee demonstrated.

"They're so expensive. . . ."

"Mum, you should get one," Daniel said. "I think it'll really make a difference."

The employee cleared his throat. "Actually, we don't have any in stock right now."

I felt like I was given a reprieve.

The employee smiled. "But you can reserve one." When I hesitated, he assured me, "You wouldn't be making a commitment to buy it."

I looked at Daniel and shrugged; it couldn't hurt. I knew I probably wouldn't buy it.

I forgot about it until a couple of days later, when Daniel asked me if it had arrived. I checked my e-mail. Not yet. The next day, I checked again. Nothing.

I was on the phone to my parents the following day. "I've been considering buying an e-reader. They're a bit expensive, and I'm not really sure that it'll do the trick—"

I was taken aback when Mum interrupted me. "We'll pay for it. Buy it."

And I was even more surprised when Dad added, "And don't get the cheaper one. This is important."

When I got off the phone, I told Daniel about their reaction. "Maybe you're right; maybe it *is* a good idea."

He rolled his eyes at me.

I received the e-mail notification at 11:00 p.m. on a Wednesday: it had to be picked up by Friday. The store was closed on Thursday—it was Thanksgiving. On Friday morning, I was standing outside the store as it opened.

That evening, I curled up in bed and started reading. At one point, I paused briefly. *It's getting late. I'll just finish this first chapter.* When I reached the end of the chapter, I discovered that I'd actually completed three chapters.

I had been immersed in the story. I had become one of the characters in the book. I hadn't enjoyed a book this much since . . . since the bleeds. I had forgotten how rich an experience reading could be.

But why is this working? Why didn't the large-print books work for me?

I looked down at the page. Actually, it was the equivalent of a quarter of a page in a real book; there was not enough space on the screen to display an entire page. *Of course!* Not only can print size cause difficulties in reading, but so can the amount of information on the page.

Once again, I am a voracious reader. I resort to reading "real" books only when there is no other option, when the book is unavailable for downloading onto my e-reader. Of course, that works only for easy-reading books.

The textbook for Matrices was not available for the e-reader, and it wasn't easy reading.

I discussed my frustrations over the lack of an e-book version with Judy.

"According to the Americans with Disabilities Act, they have to accommodate your needs. I'm sure we can figure out a solution." Judy had been an advocate for kids with special needs, especially those whose disabilities weren't obvious to the casual observer.

We had special needs students at Carnegie Mellon; as teachers, we had to accommodate them. I contacted our office for disability resources and explained my situation.

Larry, the manager, asked, "So, you just need the print enlarged? If we scan the textbook, you'll be able to enlarge the pages."

By the end of the day, Larry had sent me scans of the entire book. I was elated. All my fears shrank and receded into the background; the dread vanished. Until I opened one of the files he'd sent.

When I magnified it sufficiently for my needs, I encountered a problem I had not anticipated: the page didn't fit on my computer screen. When I scrolled side to side as I read each line, I lost continuity and my issues with short-term memory kicked in—I couldn't remember one end of the line by the time I scrolled to the start of the next line. And after I'd read a few sentences, the side-to-side motion set off vertigo. Simply enlarging the type was not the solution.

In the meantime, Judy tracked down information about obtaining a digital version of the book from the publisher. Clearly, this was a more viable option. I looked up the publisher's website and was relieved to discover that the procedure for obtaining a digital version was relatively straightforward. I just needed to fill out a couple of forms and have Larry sign off on my request.

I filled out the forms and forwarded the information to Larry, asking that he send the publisher an e-mail verifying the legitimacy of my request. Then I waited. And waited. And waited.

I understood that the publisher, cautious about copyright infringement issues, had to make sure that everything was kosher before it released a digital version. I was aware that the process could take a while. But I started early, more than two months before the class would begin, and I wasn't concerned. I knew that I'd get the book in plenty of time. Even if it took a whole month, I'd be fine.

But a month later, I began getting nervous. What if I didn't get it in time for the beginning of the semester? When another week went by, my anxiety escalated. What if the publisher declined my request outright?

Finally, two weeks before classes started, after a few misfires, misunderstandings, and several nudging e-mails on my part, I had access to the digital version. I was both relieved and uneasy. What if I had to relearn a lot of material? Would I have enough time to prepare myself?

I downloaded the file, opened to the first chapter, and flew through it. I sampled a later chapter, then another.

I texted Cindy: "Woohoo! I can read the digital version of

the textbook! I understand it!" I e-mailed Judy and phoned Joyce with the good news, too.

I was back in the running. I knew I was ready to teach the course successfully—theory, proofs, and all.

I stared at my student unseeing, my mind a blank—utter silence, inky-black darkness, no words, no thoughts, no emotions. I blinked and felt the hum as my brain rebooted and the lights in my circuitry blinked back on, one by one.

Once all my systems were operational, I became aware of my student, still staring at me, waiting for a response. I recalled his question and searched the math files in my mind for an answer, but my brain wouldn't cooperate.

I blinked again and shook my head, as if to clear it, and apologized. "Sorry about that. I seem to have fallen through a hole in my brain."

I'd just concluded an evening review session. Even before my life turned upside down, I found evening sessions exhausting. Once they were over, dredging up any pearls of wisdom for the stragglers was hard work. Now, post-brain injury, the difficulty is tenfold: I have to draw from my reserves to do anything in the evening, let alone teaching, and by the end of class, I feel completely spent. It is as if there are no pearls of wisdom left. What used to be a brief moment of blankness now endures for what feels like a lifetime.

Since I returned to teaching after the brain surgeries, by the end of one class, I'm wiped out. After the second, I feel like a babbling idiot. I can't make sense of questions that students throw at me, and when I finally do make the necessary connections, I have trouble accessing answers, then trouble finding the words for my responses. What in the past would have been a brief "senior moment" now lasts longer. In reality, it's usually no more than a few minutes, but to me, a person who used to be an extremely fast thinker, it seems like an eternity.

This semester was much worse than usual, much more draining. Since my workload was heavier than it had ever been, even compared with the pre-brain injury era, it would have been hard enough to teach the humanities courses. Teaching the more advanced Matrices course made it all that much harder.

Everything seemed to be working against me.

I made a serious error in the way I chose to manage my time. I knew that my effectiveness in the classroom correlated with the amount of rest I got. I mistakenly believed that I would be better off having all my teaching-related duties clumped together, to allow me to maximize my time at home, where I could rest. So, given the choice, I opted to teach my classes back to back, with no break to recover and regroup, and I held my office hours directly after my second class. On top of that, in my extreme anxiety about teaching the higher-level course, I doubled my usual prep time before each lecture.

Adding to the drain on my systems was the fact that I could not rest after office hours were over. Instead, I mentally reviewed my classroom and office-hours performance. I reexamined each proof, each example, each answer to every question, wondering if I could have improved on my explanations.

I gave excellent, well-thought-out lectures; my explanations were clear, my slides well organized, informative, and uncluttered. I proceeded through the lectures at an optimal pace for the students, neither too slow nor too fast.

However, teaching is not just about presentations. It is also about interacting with students, both personally and academically, and that's where I failed miserably.

I was utterly exhausted, both physically and emotionally, especially on days that I taught. And, of course, when fatigue struck, so did the bloody brain, exacerbating neurological deficits. Also, unable to submit to the bloody brain's demands for rest, it punished me with severe headaches, which added to my difficulties. My memory was affected, I had trouble accessing vocabulary, and the rate at which I thought was slow.

I should have been able to respond to questions and comments more clearly and in a timelier fashion. Several times, I had to get back to students with an answer after class was over. In addition, I lacked the energy and wherewithal to draw the students out; I had a lot of trouble making personal connections with them, and that detracted from the learning environment.

Before this semester, as I'd strived to perform on the job, I'd often floundered as I struggled to stay afloat while trying to maintain a decent quality of life. Now, I was drowning.

I realize I could not have paced myself any better than I did. I cut back on activities in my personal life in order to survive, I tried to stay home to rest one day a week, I did my best to take naps on my off-teaching days in order to replenish my sorely depleted energy reserves. But it was not enough—and there was nothing more I could have done.

I understand that not all losses can be compensated for, not all obstacles can be surmounted by hard work and stubbornness, not all problems can be fixed. But understanding doesn't make me feel any less like a failure. It doesn't lessen my grief and despair over my inability to overcome my limitations.

I'm angry, too. I should have followed my instincts. I should have been more assertive and refused to teach the course.

I am also afraid, still filled with anxiety.

According to my neuropsychologist, I have the ability, the brain power, but I have lost facility, speed. Despite my neuropsychologist's assurance that I have lost little brain power, like many brain injury survivors, I cannot help but question my ability. Even if my schedule had been more favorable, even if I had not suffered from fatigue and headaches, would I really have done significantly better?

Could this happen again in the future? Can I still think of myself as a mathematician? Do I still belong in the mathematical sciences department at Carnegie Mellon University? Should I be thinking of going on medical disability?

chapter twenty-five

2008–2013:
Pain

TWO-FIFTEEN A.M.

Two Tylenol, three Advil.

The distant sound of a train's air horn saws through my brain. A ragged laceration trails every muffled bellow. I try to relax; my head sinks into the pillow, and as I yawn, pain rips through my head.

The combination of sleep and meds is my only chance. I have to ease the tension in my mind and body. I lie motionless, my muscles loose, my eyes closed, breathing evenly, my thoughts drifting from one random image to another: swaying on the hammock on the shore of Lake Izabal, watching the water; strolling on the beach with my father, looking back at the waves lapping at our footprints. The images flow lazily through my mind, but my escalating headache advances, casting a dark shadow, blotting them out.

Reading might make me sleepy but might intensify the headache. The pain is already excruciating—I won't notice the difference. However, sleep might actually cure the headache.

I read and read, but drowsiness eludes me. There is only jagged pain. Pain defines me. Pain is everything. Every movement batters. Every thought pounds.

4:03.

Two hours, twelve minutes before I can pop more painkillers.

Time passes, or not. Pain is all I know.

Images lumber through my mind: Bill trudging up the stairs;
hiking with Joyce through the woods; riding my tricycle up a
steep hill.

I struggle to open my eyes. I turn my head toward the clock.
I move slowly, wincing as I go.

7:17. An hour's safety margin.

In order to minimize the chances of hemorrhages from the remaining angiomas, the neurologists in Arizona warned me to
stay away from painkillers with blood-thinning properties, such
as ibuprofen and aspirin. They also told me to avoid Imitrex, a
migraine medication that narrows blood vessels in the head. I
left the hospital with a prescription for Tylenol with codeine.
Not only did it lose all potency within a month, it also caused
increasing problems with my digestive system. I reacted to Vi-
codin the same way.

I settled on Tylenol without codeine, but after a while, it lost
its effectiveness, too.

The only pain meds available to me that still make a difference are the ones I'm not supposed to take, the ones that contain ibuprofen. But even those, at best, dull the edges for a little
while, merely postponing the brunt of the headache.

I don't like taking painkillers, and it's not clear that they're
worth the general feeling of malaise they cause. More and more,
I let my headaches run their course, without pharmaceutical
intervention, especially if I can afford to spend a good few hours

in bed. If it's my brain's way of forcing me to rest, I should comply and rest, if at all possible.

I use meds only when I need to keep going, and then, I resort to combinations that include ibuprofen. There are no other options.

I lie in bed in a haze of pain. I must do something. But my thinking is foggy. I push thoughts through the smog. Two Tylenol and . . . how many Advil? Three? Four? Five? Three did nothing. Will four work? They usually do. But sometimes not. Five? Five always feels wrong. Three Tylenol? My gorge rises. Not an option. Two Aleve? I gag. Definitely not.

Perhaps there's no point. But I have so much to do. I have to teach. One more try?

The bell at the railroad crossing bings in the distance, tearing through my universe again, and again, and again.

Three Aleve.

chapter twenty-six

2008−2013:

Moods and Meds

W AS IT LONELINESS?
Joyce was still in England, and the kids were
with Bill. The trip to Santa Fe with Cindy was beyond wonderful; it was a wrench to return to real life.

Perhaps loneliness explained the tears.

But I usually love having time to myself. Also, Joyce travels a
lot and the kids are with Bill every other week, and it'd been ten
days since I'd said good-bye to Cindy. I should have been over
the worst of it by now. I hadn't been this weepy under similar
circumstances in the past. Or had I? I couldn't remember; perhaps I had.

Lonely or not, I certainly wasn't at a level that warranted
meltdowns.

What about hormonal issues?

Given that I was perimenopausal and my cycle fairly erratic,
it was hard to judge. I studied the calendar with a critical eye.

I'd been fragile ever since I'd returned from Santa Fe, more
than a week ago. PMS could account for only a couple of days
at best.

So it wasn't hormones.

What else could bring on such wretchedness?

My tears during the *Harry Potter* movie didn't raise any red flags—Joyce told me that she'd cried, too. Weeping over the news about my friend Mickey was not unexpected, either. I wasn't alone in my grief. The news wasn't good: her cancer was back, and . . . it just wasn't good.

I started becoming suspicious after a week of emotional vulnerability. Tears welled up several times a day, every day, over trouble finding a pen, over forgetting to buy toothpaste, over nothing.

What could it be?

A vague memory tugged at my consciousness: I'd been through something similar before, a more dramatic version. It was a long time ago, it brought misery and hopelessness . . . and then it clicked: the meds.

I recognized the emotional pattern, the unwarranted tears and the despair, from those first six months after the surgeries. I remembered how much better I felt after my psychiatrist increased my dosage of Lamictal. Now I was experiencing exactly the same type of turmoil, and the timing matched when I'd begun taking a lower daily dose—the day after I'd come home from the trip to Santa Fe.

My neurologist, suspecting epilepsy, put me on Lamictal in May 2007. I'd ramped up to 300 milligrams per day, in increments of 50 milligrams. And after I'd spent a week or so at 300 milligrams per day, the frequency of the seizures had lessened, until they'd ended altogether a couple of weeks later.

I was seizure free for over three months, until the evening after the first surgery. On August 8, 2007, I experienced a tonic-clonic, or grand mal, seizure. After I suffered a couple more seizures soon after that, the hospital neurologists increased my dose of Lamictal to 350 milligrams and added 1,500 milligrams of another antiseizure med, Keppra.

After I'd taken a couple of doses, I knew something didn't feel right. I was not sure why—there was no concrete evidence of bad side effects—but somehow the Keppra felt wrong, very wrong. I refused to take any more. The neurologists argued with me quite vehemently, but I, too, was vehement—I would not take the Keppra, no matter what. They surrendered and increased the Lamictal to 400 milligrams.

Back home, I was sure that my neurologist would lower the Lamictal back to 300 milligrams when I went to see him for my first postsurgery follow-up appointment. I'd never been completely comfortable taking any dosage of the Lamictal. I was wary of antiseizure meds, concerned about side effects. What else was it doing to my brain? To my body?

I understood why the hospital neurologists had raised the dose. I had reluctantly accepted it because I assumed it was temporary. I was under the impression that the seizures I'd experienced in the hospital were caused by the surgical trauma to my brain. I believed that once I was a few weeks beyond the surgeries—plenty of time for my brain to have recovered from the trauma—there'd be no reason to expect a recurrence of the seizures. In fact, I assumed that the threat of any form of seizures was over now that the angiomas had been removed and the brain surgeries were a thing of the past. I was finally on the road to recovery, sure that within five years, probably less, I'd be off the Lamictal altogether.

It never occurred to me that within a few months I'd be taking a higher dose. And I certainly never imagined that the mood-stabilizing property of the antiseizure meds would be the reason for the increase. I'd have been shocked if anyone had suggested that I'd have issues with depression, or, even worse, that I'd end up taking meds to manage depression.

Four months after the surgeries, when I became suicidal and finally recognized my need for antidepressants, my psychiatrist increased my Lamictal dose to 600 milligrams.

I responded well to the increase; my emotional state improved immensely. I was back in control of myself, back to being myself. Most of the time. My tears were confined to the handful of days each month when I was ovulating and when I had PMS.

Given my continual discomfort about meds, that handful of days seemed like a small price to pay for staying with Lamictal, rather than experimenting with other, possibly more problematic meds.

Over the next year, the depression diminished. I no longer felt that same teary-eyed vulnerability, not even during those few difficult days within each menstrual cycle. My memory of all that despair and devastation faded, and I started thinking seriously about trying to decrease the dosage of the Lamictal.

I'd always kept my use of any type of medication to a minimum: painkillers for headaches and antibiotics for bacterial infections, nothing else. And now here I was, popping pills daily— three shield-shaped, peach colored pills for seizures and depression; two oval, periwinkle-blue pills for blood pressure, to prevent headaches and minimize the chances of additional bleeds; two round, light blue pills for a folic-acid deficiency.

Taking all those pills bothered me. I couldn't get used to it; I felt like I was poisoning myself, and the Lamictal was the worst of the lot.

Several brain injury survivors who'd been on antiseizure meds had told me that coming off the meds was like donning new glasses—the clarity and focus were astonishing. They said that you don't realize that you've been living in a fog until the meds are out of your system.

After Sarah, as a baby, had been sleeping through the night for a while, I discovered that a research paper I'd been working on since I was pregnant with her was riddled with errors. No longer sleep-deprived, I was not only aware of the mistakes but also able to fix them quite easily. I remember rejoicing in my return to my old, thinking self, wondering how I could not have noticed how befogged I'd been all that time.

Was Lamictal blurring the world to me? I didn't feel as if I were living in a fog. But how would I know unless I lowered the dose?

I wanted to live with as much clarity as possible. I would have loved to eventually come off the Lamictal completely. But by now, I was aware that that might never happen.

Even though I believed I had not experienced any seizures since my hospital stay, I was not willing to take chances. A single seizure would cause a dramatic change in my life. One seizure would prevent me from driving. I'd have to move out of the suburbs. I'd probably have to quit dragon boating because of the location. Visiting the kids in college would be extremely difficult. I was willing to do anything to eliminate all risk of seizures, even if it meant that I would have to take meds indefinitely. I could live with staying on 300 milligrams daily, if necessary.

The 300 milligrams held a special significance for me. It was my starting dose, the dose that my neurologist prescribed to combat seizures alone, my dose going into the surgeries.

I was convinced that the sole reason for the depression was the surgeries. In my mind, any dosage above 300 milligrams targeted the depression and had nothing to do with seizures. I hoped that one day, as part of my recovery from the surgeries, I'd be depression free, no longer needing meds. I believed that

I'd already made enormous strides in that direction. After all, I hadn't felt depressed in more than a year. It didn't occur to me that the higher Lamictal levels had anything to do with that.

My headaches were another reason for my wanting to decrease the Lamictal.

The blood pressure medication, verapamil, which my neurologist prescribed when I was first diagnosed with cavernous angiomas, was supposed to minimize the chances of brain hemorrhages. At the same time, he hoped that it would prevent my migraines. It did not forestall the hemorrhages, but it did cure the migraines. After the bleeds, I started experiencing frequent explosive headaches, far worse than migraines.

At first, I was convinced that these headaches were a consequence of the brain injury, but after taking 600 milligrams of Lamictal per day for a while, I began wondering if the two were related. Headaches are listed as one of the possible side effects. Could the meds be exacerbating the headaches, if not actually causing them? I wasn't sure, but, given their severity, I was ready to grasp at anything that might help. Perhaps a lower dose of Lamictal would decrease the frequency and intensity of the headaches.

A couple of years after the surgeries, my psychiatrist permitted me to cut down to 500 milligrams per day. Lowering the dose made me feel as if I were headed toward a full recovery from the brain injury, or at least close to a full recovery.

The decrease did affect me psychologically—depression made a comeback. But it was not debilitating, and the worst of it was limited to a few days each menstrual cycle, as it had been during the first year postsurgery. Physically, I saw no improvement; the headaches persisted.

After a few months, the depression eased up, and I was ready to reduce the dose further.

Both my neurologist and my psychiatrist allowed me to lower the dose again, to 450 milligrams. I stayed on 450 milligrams for approximately six months and then dropped down once more, to 400 milligrams.

I had no difficulties over the transitions from 500 to 400 milligrams. My depression remained under control. But the headaches persisted.

A few days before I was to take a trip with Cindy to Santa Fe, four years since the surgeries, my neurologist cleared me for an additional decrease in the dose, to 300 milligrams, though he seemed a bit apprehensive and asked that I report to him in a couple of months.

At Cindy's request, I waited until after our trip to make any adjustments. But by the time I returned home, I lost the connection—I forgot why the neurologist and Cindy had been concerned about the change and why I'd agreed to wait. As soon as I got back from Santa Fe, I dropped directly from 400 to 300 milligrams.

At the 400 milligrams level, I'd been taking 200 milligrams twice a day. When I decreased my dosage of Lamictal to 300 milligrams daily, I followed my neurologist's advice: I took 100 milligrams in the morning and 200 milligrams in the evening. It made sense; taking the lower dose in the morning would minimize the impact of the side effects. In particular, if the Lamictal was indeed blanketing me in a fog, I'd rather it did so while I was asleep than during my waking hours.

I was thrilled. I was finally back to 300 milligrams, proof positive that the emotional effects of the brain injury were behind me.

I sobbed, devastated, over . . . was it about a sink full of dirty dishes? Or that my teammate, Peggy, hadn't said hi to me at practice? All I remember is that it was something minor. Later in the day, I felt overwhelmed by despair as I recalled Mickey's acting distant when I'd last seen her.

I tried to reason it out.

It wasn't loneliness. It probably wasn't PMS—that usually didn't last more than a day or so, and the whole week had been wretched. It had been since I'd returned from Santa Fe. . . .

It had to be the change in the meds.

But wait: Did that really make sense? I had no trouble reducing from 500 to 450 to 400 milligrams. Why was the drop to 300 milligrams problematic? Was it just too quick?

Despite having spiraled downward for several weeks, I was reluctant to bump up the dosage from the magic 300 milligrams. Anyway, I wasn't convinced that I was at too low a daily dose— the issue was probably the abrupt decrease. I'd kept the evening dose at 200 milligrams. The 100 milligrams in the morning was the likely culprit.

Anxious to stick with that all-important number, I switched to taking 150 milligrams in the morning and 150 milligrams at night, hoping that shifting to a higher morning dose would dampen the daytime depression. Within a couple of days, I started feeling better, but I wanted to give it a while longer before I celebrated.

A week passed, and I was still doing well. It felt right; I'd obviously found the solution.

But PMS sent me plummeting downward, and I didn't come back up.

Depression started to interfere with my work. I couldn't face some straightforward aspects of my job, like responding to emails from my students or signing letters of recommendation. It affected my behavior, too, especially my interactions with other people.

When Cindy asked me why I was so angry with her, it shocked me into the realization that I'd become impatient and irritable, not only with her, but also with Sarah. My relationship with Sarah was a bit rocky already; I didn't want to jeopardize it any further. I needed to protect my relationship with my teenage daughter and with my friends. I needed to raise the dose to 350 milligrams.

I was originally going to wait for my appointment with my psychiatrist before I upped my dose of Lamictal, but the semester was beginning. I had to be able to function, and I couldn't in my current emotional state. I decided to increase my morning dose to 200 milligrams and leave the evening dose as it was, at 150 milligrams, for a total of 350 milligrams per day.

The next morning, I took 200 milligrams.

I was sure this was the answer. This way, I was back on track with reducing the dosage from 400 by 50 milligrams at a time. Perhaps my body would need some time to adjust, perhaps I'd have to put up with some fragility a few days per month for a while, but I was okay with that. I'd gone through that before. It was doable.

The fluctuations in my estrogen levels during a normal menstrual cycle amplified the symptoms of depression, so I would need a higher dose of Lamictal to keep the amplified symptoms in check. However, given the time lag between when I popped a pill and when it took effect, combined with the unpredictability of my perimenopausal menstrual cycle, it was not logistically possible to adjust the level of Lamictal to match my evolving moods throughout my cycle. I needed to discover the minimum dose that would keep me away from the edge at all times.

I wanted to believe that 350 milligrams per day was that dose.

I am afraid of becoming suicidal. I recognize the warning signs, the hopelessness, the desolation, the feeling that I am a burden on people who care for me. No, I am not there, yet. Not today. But I am too close to the edge. I am afraid that a mere nudge could tip me over.

It's all been too much. The beginning of this academic year has been extremely stressful, practicing parallel parking with Sarah and dealing with the aftermath of her repeatedly failing driving tests has not been easy, and dragon boating has been less than joyful at times. I just found out that the largest of my remaining angiomas has caused seizures in the past, which contradicts my doctors' repeated assurances that it was of no concern. And the continuing struggle with the meds . . . just too much. Then today . . .

I spent most of the day crying. I did manage to put on my public face when necessary. I wore my supportive-mother mask for Sarah's latest failure at the driver's licensing center. I displayed my smiling teacher's mask during a meeting with my students. Luckily, when the mask slipped and my eyes filled with tears, no one noticed. Sarah was too wrapped up in her own disappointment to notice, and the students couldn't see—they sat too far away from me. Once my public appearances were over, there was nothing to prevent the tears.

The latest devastation was over a misunderstanding with Cindy. Both of us are emotional people, and every great once in a while, we reach resonance. Today was one of those days. We were both feeling vulnerable, Cindy probably because she was physically exhausted, and I because I have been fragile for weeks. She thought I was upset with her, which upset her, which in turn upset me, and it escalated from there.

I used to think that I could never take my own life. No—I used to *know* that I could never take my own life. But after the brain hemorrhages, I learned that there are no guarantees. I had been suicidal and could become so again.

I phoned Cindy several times during the day, trying to work through the barrage of emotions that tore through us. After one of our exchanges, I sank low enough to wish that taking a temporary break from life were possible. Not a permanent break, not suicide, but perhaps something akin to a nervous breakdown.

My mind veered away from the thought. I could not, would not go there. Those reflections were far too close to thoughts of suicide. I will not let myself go there again.

I am afraid that I'll be swallowed by the maw that is suicide—not right now, but maybe later today, or tomorrow, the day after. I know 350 milligrams is not enough.

At 300 and 350 milligrams, I endured no more than two, possibly three, headaches, and none of them sent me crawling into bed.

If I increase the Lamictal to 400 milligrams, will the frequent, debilitating headaches return?

"I agree, you do need to go back up to the four hundred milligrams per day." After a brief hesitation, my psychiatrist added, "You may have to go higher."

I gulped and nodded. I knew she was right. I couldn't afford to be as near the edge as I had been the previous week.

Given how badly hormonal changes affect my depression,

and given how unpredictable those changes have become as I undergo perimenopause, I know that I cannot make any assumptions. I don't know what other surprises perimenopause holds for me. I don't know when menopause will release me from this nightmare, or whether it will release me. There is no way to foresee the outcome.

I have to be realistic. I have to face the fact that my depression could worsen, which could indeed mean additional increases in my Lamictal dose.

The higher dose dramatically improved my mood.

The headaches returned in full force.

Headaches versus depression? I'll take the headaches any day.

A few months later, I had to increase the dosage to 450 milligrams per day. And within a few days, I started feeling like myself once again. But I wasn't ready to celebrate; it was too early. I wanted to wait and see.

It's been about six months now. I still feel like myself.

Will it last? Will I have to increase the dose further?

chapter twenty-seven

2008–2013:
Fear and the Memory of Fear

'M AFRAID TO MOVE.

There's nothing out there for me, nothing to hold me, no support. I cannot surrender myself to the endless void.

I was hanging on to the tent pole, gripping it hard with both hands, for what—ten, fifteen minutes? More? It was my lifeline, the only thing that made sense in the mindless chaos surrounding me, the only thing that kept me from being swept into bedlam. Patches of colors encircled me, ever moving, shifting, lurching, staggering. Words, laughter, rumbles, bellows, shrieks darted by. The only object that maintained its solidity was the tent pole.

Joyce's voice emerged from the madness. "Let's get you out of here."

I heard the words rumble, but they did not register. They came from outside the precarious haven of me and my tent pole. I was completely overcome by my battle for survival: my struggle to keep the world at bay, my fight to stem the flow of raw fear that flooded me.

"C'mon, let's go for a walk."

Her words grated on my consciousness.

My brain could not handle more than the bare basics. Any

input from the outside, including Joyce's voice, was more than I could fathom.

"C'mon, Deb."

A wisp of a memory, fainter than a thought, floated by: her voice meant safety. The next thought slammed directly into it: it was too late; no one could rescue me. The only safety zone I had access to was right here, me and the tent pole. There was nothing safe about "out there," where Joyce existed.

I felt her touch on my arm and teetered. I heard my breathing, quick, loud. I saw movement out of the corner of my eye and lurched away from it, then swayed back and forth, my biceps and triceps expanding and contracting as I gripped the pole, fighting to regain my unsteady equilibrium.

"You can do it."

Do what? Move away from my tent pole? But there was danger beyond it. Danger of falling, danger of . . . everything.

"I'll help you."

How? I knew she meant well, but it was far too late—it was impossible. I studied my feet. They were in constant motion, my toes wiggling up and down, my ankles wobbling from side to side, my weight continually shifting from the balls of my feet to my heels, to the sides and back, all my muscles tensing and releasing, tensing and releasing.

I couldn't go anywhere. Where would I go? Everywhere was noise and colors and motion. There was nowhere to go.

She was insistent. "C'mon. Just follow me. You can do this."

But no, I couldn't, not even with a guiding hand. I was too far-gone. There was no way out of this one. I was really stuck this time, holding on to the tent pole for dear life, held captive by the sheer, intense fear of losing myself to the chaos, multiplied by the fear of an eternal fall.

"Take one step over here."

She grasped me firmly by the arm. I rocked wildly on my feet. Gradually, the rocking abated, and with it, the worst of the fear began to subside. My body settled back into the constant perturbations and adjustments that kept me upright.

A realization emerged through my defenses—Joyce's hold on me had dampened my oscillations. Her support felt sturdier than the tent pole's. It was safer. I realized that I could lean on her. I should lean on her. I should let go of the tent pole . . . if only I could move.

I contemplated my feet. I focused hard, willing my right foot to shift toward Joyce. I tried to put more weight on my right heel, but my foot rebelled, causing my entire body to lurch to the left, back toward the tent pole, away from Joyce. My grip on the pole tightened.

Joyce moved in closer, her body right up against mine, solid, safe, her left arm around me, the other supporting my right arm. She tugged slightly at it, and again my body rocked sideways in response; I heard myself take short, shallow breaths.

"Steady, steady. I've got you."

I felt my eyes smart. It was hopeless. I was now mentally able to accept her help—in theory, I could acknowledge Joyce's existence and let her into my world, but in practice, my brain couldn't function at that level—I couldn't do my part in the rescue operation.

I gulped and concentrated on my feet. If I turned toward her, I'd be fine. All I needed to do was turn both feet in her direction. I tried to gather my wayward wits to focus on that one tiny action. I tried to do it in one motion, shift both feet at the same time. My wobbling feet weren't complying. Perhaps one foot would suffice. . . .

Before I finished the thought, something happened. *Did Joyce pull me? Did I somehow manage to move?*

I was suddenly in Joyce's arms, fully supported, my head buried in her shoulder, my shoulders shaking as I sobbed.

Joyce held me quietly, sheltering me from the rest of the world. Some time later, I realized that the sobs had quieted down to the occasional whimper, though tears still streamed. Finally, the tears dried to a mere trickle, then stopped altogether.

Joyce kept her arms around me. I noticed that my feet and calf muscles were still in constant motion, trying to compensate for my lack of balance. Joyce must have noticed as well.

"Why don't you sit down?"

I was sure it was a good idea; Joyce would not lead me astray. But it did not feel like a good idea. It felt like a terrible idea, a terrifying idea. I could not, would not, sit down.

"Here, I put the chair right behind you. Just sit down."

I couldn't—I would fall, forever.

I pondered my feet. Did I dare I move them? Was I even capable of . . .

She—*she*—was forcing me down!

A wave of terror swamped me. My heart raced; my pulse pounded in my ears in rhythm with my gasping breaths as I hyperventilated. I was falling into a vacuum, into eternity, into the world I didn't dare acknowledge, let alone trust.

A lifetime later, the canvas of my folding chair cradled me, but fear still consumed me.

My chest heaving, my body shaking, I hunkered down, hunched over, the brim of my baseball cap hiding me from the world, hiding the world from me.

I'm hungry. As I think about food, saliva accumulates in my mouth. I swallow, except I don't. I can't. I try again. I work my throat but can't quite complete the action. *What the*—*?* I try again, focusing hard. It works, eventually, with difficulty. I experiment and try to swallow again. Nope. Not happening. I work my tongue, the muscles in the back of my mouth, my throat. Nothing.

Another bleed? No, it can't . . . But this is new; what else could it be? I've never had trouble swallowing. Not even in the hospital.

Or have I? I think back. I have had difficulty swallowing several times since the surgeries. But until now, I've always somehow, with hard work and complete focus, managed to overcome the difficulty; I've never actually been totally incapable of swallowing.

I try again. Nothing. I remind myself to breathe.

A brain stem injury can cause difficulty swallowing. A friend's niece who underwent brain stem surgery wasn't discharged from the hospital until she overcame the problem. Another friend of mine had a husband who choked to death because he couldn't swallow. He was afflicted with Alzheimer's; it's not unusual in Alzheimer's patients.

Fear threatens to overwhelm me, like huge, dark waves gaining momentum, a tsunami in the making, speeding toward me.

More saliva accumulates, about to overflow. I try swallowing again. Almost. I almost get it. I try again, and again. I come close each time.

Fear starts evolving into terror.

My fears are primordial, rawer and much more immediate than they used to be.

I used to be afraid of heights but was able to maintain my cool and walk away. I now become petrified when a sheer drop confronts me. The ground threatens to fall away from me, and I cannot move away without help.

I often wake up in the middle of the night from nightmares, consumed by terror, unable to separate dream from reality. I have phoned Daniel in college, Sarah on sleepovers, and my parents in Israel, convinced that something terrible has happened to them, positive that my dream was real.

My heart pounds loudly at the mere threat of bumping my head when I stand at the top of a steep staircase or when I step on and off an escalator. Panic overpowers me whenever I hit my head on a cabinet door or during a fall.

I am terrified of suffering another brain injury, of any possible indication of another bleed. When people speak and all I hear is a senseless collection of words, or when my own words become tangled, I have to remind myself to breathe. I wonder, is this a new symptom? Has another angioma become symptomatic?

I am a member of the Angioma Alliance, an organization that provides information and support for angioma patients. Into my third year after the surgeries, one of their nurses mentioned that angiomas can grow back and that I could grow new ones.

My breath caught in my throat, sitting heavy, blocking my airways. She continued speaking, but I couldn't hear her over the roar in my head. When I did catch a word here and there, it sounded like gibberish.

My terror surprised me. This was not new information; my neurosurgeon had mentioned the possibility of the angiomas' growing back when I'd first met him, and I'd spoken of it to my neurologist at least twice before.

One evening, I read, "Brain injury survivors are at high risk for early-onset dementia."

How early? Next year? In ten years? Before I hit sixty? I lie in bed, my eyes wide open, staring unseeing at the ceiling.

I recoil at the imagined image of myself shuffling along, leaning on Daniel's arm, a vacant look in my eyes, a look of infinite patience in his. I shy away from thoughts of Sarah, hesitating, torn, needing to run an errand, looking back at me as I sit on the sofa, facing the front door, confused, trying to puzzle out the situation.

I blink in an attempt to rid myself of these visions, fear rising toward panic. I can't become that lost woman. I mustn't become that lost woman.

But as I lie there, the immediacy of my fears fades away; the emotional content of my thoughts fast loses its potency.

I do not live in perpetual, unrelenting terror. My factual memory is lousy; many of my memories of events rapidly dim to become, at best, faint recollections, which may or may not be resurrected with some prodding. My emotional memory is much worse; most of my memories of emotions are fleeting and cannot be resurrected.

Before the hemorrhages, my memories were enriched with emotional content. Now, it feels as if the connection between my factual and emotional memories is damaged. I sometimes remember the facts about my emotions ("I was really upset") or I extrapolate from the facts ("I must have felt really scared"). Strong emotions, such as terror or devastation, sometimes evoke memories. But few memories evoke strong emotions, and many evoke no emotions whatsoever. In all but a few cases, I am no longer capable of reliving those emotions, other than through my writing.

The fear of suffering from dementia is no more—the emotional detachment has completely taken over. It is as if all I am left with is a lifeless report about a stranger.

Next week, will I remember lying in my bed, filled with terror? Next month, will I remember that I am at high risk for early-onset dementia?

2008-2013:
Communication

A WAVE OF OVERWHELMING FATIGUE WASHES THROUGH me. *No! Not now! Not in the boat.* But I cannot outrun the wave that is about to engulf me. I manage to pull the paddle into the boat before I am swamped. My eyes close, I slump forward, my head nods onto my chest, and my hand loses its grip on the paddle and slides into the water as the systems in my brain shut down. I feel as if I am settling into the safety of a protective cocoon that envelops my mind. I've been through this enough now that I know what's happening: my brain has shut down nonessential systems while it clears my circuits.

Larry calls out. "Paddles up!"

I feel the boat jolt as my teammates whip their paddles to the ready position. "Deb! Put your paddle up!"

Jane is sitting next to me. "What's wrong? Deb! Are you okay?"

I hear the panic in her voice. I want to calm her down; I want to tell her that there's no need to worry, that I'm in a safe place, in a shutdown. I want to explain that I'll pop out of it on my own, I'll be fine, I just need a couple of minutes. But I cannot; I've lost muscle tone, and my breathing is too shallow to activate my voice.

I know that my best course of action is to relax into it. I

know that interrupting the process by fighting it would merely slow it down and cut back on its effectiveness, leaving me with residual overload, hypersensitive to subtle triggers. I nestle comfortably into my cocoon and wait for the all-clear signal. My hand trails in the water.

"Coach! We have a problem!"

No, it's okay, I'm fine. There's no need to fret. But my concerns about worrying others retreat as my mind focuses on the immediate. I revel in the sensation of pressure on my hand as the warm water flows over it. I delight in the caresses of the breeze created by the motion of the dragon boat. I luxuriate in the rhythmic rocking caused by nineteen paddles pulling through the water and whipping through the air as one.

I absentmindedly recall Larry's command to paddle back to the docks with full power. *I should help.* And I pop out of the shutdown, grab my paddle, and join in, rejoicing in the force I apply as I slam my paddle into the river and pull it through the water.

Larry's voice startles me. "Get that paddle away from her!"

"But I'm fine."

"Jane! Take. It. Away. From. Her!"

When we reach the dock, I scramble out of the boat, brushing away all offers for help, and hurry to catch up with Larry.

I want my neuropsychologist, who is also my teammate, to explain shutdowns to Larry, to confirm what I'm trying to explain to him. I am concerned that Larry won't allow me to paddle in our upcoming race, the second race of the season, in Ithaca, New York.

"It wasn't a seizure. It's not a big deal. It's just that when the sensory input gets too much, my circuits get jammed up. Then my systems shut down briefly while my circuits clear and my systems reboot. This won't happen during a race. I'm fully engaged then." I refrain from telling him that I probably overloaded in the first place because he droned on and on about technique and overwhelmed my brain with a continual inflow of data.

In a race, while the adrenaline courses through my system, my focus is complete. Concentrating on paddling, on power, on technique, gives me direction. It does not allow me to stray, to become distracted and overwhelmed by input from outside the boat. I have never suffered from overload or shut down in a race.

When I shut down, my eyes close, I lose muscle tone, my breathing slows down and softens, and I'm unable to communicate. To an observer, it looks like I've lost consciousness. But inside I am fully alive, completely aware of my surroundings, and my senses of hearing and touch are totally unimpaired.

During the first couple of years postsurgery, I often shut down after I overloaded. I gathered from my neuropsychologist that this was a mechanism my brain used to unclog my jammed circuits, to bring me relief from sensory overload. Until he explained them to me, I was afraid of shutdowns, scared that I'd become trapped forever, unable to communicate, buried alive in an unresponsive body. I was afraid that I would die within a shutdown, alone. In my fear, I fought them, trying to open my eyes, convinced that if I could only open my eyes, I'd be fine.

After I discussed them with my neuropsychologist, I started welcoming them. Instead of seeing them as a tomb threatening to bury me, I saw them as a form of protection from the overpowering onslaught of data while my brain sorted itself out.

These shutdowns began happening a couple of months after the surgeries. They followed the same profile as my presurgery "seizure-like" episodes. Given the similarities between the presurgery and postsurgery episodes, I suspected that they were the same type of event. And when my neuropsychologist, who had witnessed a couple of my postsurgery spells, named them "shutdowns," I realized that all along, both before and after the surgeries, all these episodes I'd been experiencing were in fact just that.

The term "shutdown," which did not include the word "seizure," allowed me to address the on-call neurologist's diagnosis.

I now agreed with her pronouncement that they were not honest-to-goodness epileptic seizures. After all, they did not correspond to abnormal EEGs. On the other hand, contrary to her diagnosis, they were not pseudoseizures, either. They were shutdowns, another type of event, completely unrelated to seizures or any other phenomenon with a label containing the word "seizure."

Larry and I were walking side by side, heading toward the parking lot. As we were about to part ways, I said, "You realize that shutdowns aren't seizures?"

He headed in the direction of the yacht club and tossed over his shoulder, "Seizures, shutdowns—same difference."

But how could he say that? They are totally different. Aren't they?

I valued and respected Larry's opinion, and I couldn't ignore his comment. I tried to view shutdowns through his eyes. That's when it hit me: from Larry's perspective, or from the perspective of any bystander, for that matter, in terms of the outcome, there really *was* no difference. Both seizures and shutdowns were completely incapacitating.

Were the presurgery episodes in fact seizures? Were the presurgery episodes and the shutdowns really one and the same? Were shutdowns seizures?

Not all seizures are epileptogenic—a nonepileptic seizure (NES) resembles an epileptic seizure but does not involve abnormal electrical discharges in the brain.

NESs fall into two categories: psychogenic and physiologic. The triggers for physiologic NESs include consuming too much alcohol, lack of sleep, hypoglycemia, and low blood pressure. Psychogenic NESs, on the other hand, are associated with stress, anxiety, or trauma. The literature often refers to psychogenic seizures as pseudoseizures. Unfortunately, some neurologists, including the on-call neurologist at the ER, think of them as fake seizures, calls for attention.

I knew that I was not faking my balance issues. The bloody brain was real. The bleeds were a fact. The symptoms had to be real; they felt real. This nightmare was not all in my mind. I was not mentally ill. These episodes were not pseudo-anything. When my neurologist prescribed antiseizure meds and the seizure-like episodes stopped plaguing me soon thereafter, it was a clear indication that they were in fact epileptic seizures—real seizures.

Epileptic seizures are split into several categories and subcategories.

Partial seizures originate in only one part of the brain. Generalized seizures, which can be preceded by partial seizures, involve the entire brain.

Simple partial seizures do not affect awareness or memory. Depending on exactly where in the brain the seizures originate, they can cause a wide range of symptoms, including a vague feeling of detachment from the environment, a sensation of tingling, an altered sense of hearing, inability to speak, a sense of spatial distortion, convulsions, and overall muscle weakness. The events I suffered before the surgeries were consistent with symptoms of simple partial seizures and were diagnosed as such by at least one neurologist.

Complex partial seizures include loss of awareness. Often the patient has no memory of the event. Like simple partial seizures, complex partial seizures can manifest in a variety of ways: a blank stare, lip smacking, walking, and other repetitive movements. Simple partial seizures can act as lead-ins to complex partial seizures, sometimes in the form of an aura that patients frequently regard as the warning that a seizure is imminent.

All types of generalized seizures involve loss of consciousness and, like partial seizures, also vary. Tonic-clonic seizures, such as the ones I suffered in the hospital in Arizona, entail muscle stiffening and jerking, or convulsions. In atonic seizures, there is loss of muscle tone. During absence seizures, the patient blanks out and is unaware and unresponsive.

At one point, Bill insisted to the doctor that I did lose awareness during the presurgery episodes. Given that I was unresponsive and slumped over and my eyes were closed, I can understand an observer believing that I was unconscious. Would I have been aware that I'd lost awareness? Surely I would have noticed a break in the flow of the activities around me during an episode. Having followed entire conversations throughout the duration of these events, able to join in smoothly once the episodes were over, I was certain that I remained fully conscious. Of course, it is possible that I missed breaks in the flow during some of the episodes.

But why did Bill contradict me so adamantly? When I pointed out that he wasn't even there during most of the epi-

sodes, he amended his statement by saying that I'd lost awareness at least twice.

Bill's assertions led to a diagnosis of complex partial seizures.

I was kneeling by the file cabinet, frozen, my heart pumping
loudly, staring blankly at the file lying open in my hands. After a
long moment, the heavy fog that had descended on me dispersed and the words emerged back into focus.

The file I was poring over was a medical report evaluating
some of the seizures I'd endured while I was in the hospital in
Arizona. I'd been searching through my medical records for information, trying to shed light on all the various episodes I'd
experienced since the hemorrhages.

According to the report, the EEG "showed right occipital
spikes." The neurologists conjectured that the angioma in the
right occipital lobe caused the spikes. That particular angioma is
the largest of those remaining in my brain. It is about the size of
a marble; the others are tiny, the size of small ball bearings. I
knew that the neurologists were concerned about the one in the
right occipital lobe. I thought they were monitoring it because of
its size. But perhaps the reason was that it had been symptomatic.

Had it bled? I knew that if so, the chances of its bleeding
again were . . . what? Doubled? I couldn't remember the statistics. It didn't matter—I knew the chances were much higher. On
the other hand, perhaps it hadn't bled. Angiomas do not have to
bleed to cause neurological symptoms. Whether it bled or not, if
it was symptomatic once, it could become symptomatic again.
Perhaps it had been generating abnormal brain activity all this
time.

Seizures can take extremely subtle forms. Several times I lost all familiarity with my surroundings for second or two—were those seizures? What about the times when I felt a loose thread tickling the back of my calf when there was no such thread? What if seizures were still occurring and I was unaware of them?

I couldn't understand why no one saw fit to tell me. Did the doctors think I had no need to know? Bill certainly knew. He read through those medical reports carefully. Why did he withhold that information from me? Did he think he was being protective?

I understand that at times I was not physically able to handle information. But there were plenty of other opportunities to share it with me—I'd gone four years assuming that the angioma in my right occipital lobe had been asymptomatic.

I trolled the internet for information on shutdowns but found nothing. I asked my neuropsychologist for references in the professional literature.

He was emphatic: my shutdowns were bona fide neurological events, seizure events, *seizures*.

Why did my doctors have so much trouble diagnosing my presurgical episodes? Why were they always referred to as seizure-like episodes? Why did I have to wait so long to find out that my shutdowns were in fact seizures?

In my ignorance of medical issues, I often didn't even know what questions to ask, and I wasn't assertive enough to insist on clarification.

When a student in my class asks me an ill-formulated question, I investigate further. It is my responsibility to take the time and make the effort to question the student to determine the source of his or her confusion. When I feel that I understand the issue, I explain it in different ways until I am certain that I have indeed clarified the problem.

During the presurgery era, I did not encounter a single doctor who consistently did the same for me.

Too many doctors fail to ensure clarity of communication, possibly because of lack of time, lack of patience, lack of empathy, lack of respect, or a combination thereof. As a result of ineffective doctor-patient communication, far too many questions are left unasked or unanswered and lead to frequent misunderstandings with potentially dire consequences.

Before the surgeries, during my many ER visits and subsequent hospital stays, other than the residents, none of the doctors spent more than five minutes—and usually less—at my bedside.

The residents took their time, taking notes during our exchanges, acting as scouts for their attending physicians, reporting back to them. A couple of physicians were surprised by some of my answers to their questions, the same answers I gave their residents. Did the doctors distrust their residents? Or me?

The on-call neurologist who caused me so much grief was an extreme case. But she wasn't the only doctor who treated me as if my judgment were in question. A couple of others also seemed to regard my input as erroneous or irrelevant and dismissed me as if I were of no consequence.

I understand that in order to treat patients effectively, doctors probably have to distance themselves to a degree. Do some of them take it too far, to a point where they forget that we are people, too? Was this how they treated all patients, or just brain-injured ones?

2013:
Different, Not Deficient

M Y NAME IS DEBORAH BRANDON, AND I HAVE A disability.

There! I've said it, after five years. Yes, I have alluded to it in the past, but I've had difficulty actually using that word to describe myself. I *have* used it before, maybe a couple of times, but I didn't really mean it; the word popped out before I had time to think about it, in response to a question or a comment. Once it was out there, frozen, hanging in the air in front of me, I hastily averted my gaze and moved on with the conversation.

Now, I can use the word, and repeat it—*disability, disability, disability.* Now, I can stare it in the eye.

A disability is "a physical or mental condition that limits a person's movements, senses, or activities." So says the *Oxford English Dictionary.* The complete Americans with Disabilities Act definition fills pages and pages with dense legalese, including the phrase "a physical or mental impairment that substantially limits one or more of the major life activities." Indeed, my condition is mental, which causes physical issues as well, and it certainly limits one or more of my major life activities.

According to Dictionary.com, a disability is a "physical or mental handicap, especially one that prevents a person from living a full, normal life." I don't agree with the "full, normal life" part. I think that my life is pretty full, fuller than it was prior to the brain injury. As far as "normal" goes, I'm not sure I want normal. I don't think I've ever been normal.

Synonyms for "disability" include "handicap," "disadvantage," "infirmity," "impairment," "deficiency." They're not pretty, but there they are, and here I am, handicapped, infirm, deficient.

I can't bear the term "deficient."

I am not deficient. "Deficient" means "less," and I am more. I am different from how I used to be, and my days don't run as smoothly. But my days are much more colorful, and I am much more alive. More, not less.

Today, Joyce sent me upstairs to take a nap. She'd just brought me home from yet another disastrous shopping trip where I'd overloaded.

I hate this. I hate not being able to do basic tasks without help. If Joyce weren't around to pick up the slack, I'd have to hire someone. It makes me feel defeated. I hate feeling disabled.

I have not fully accepted my disability. I don't think I ever will, not completely.

But I can say the word.

chapter thirty

2013:

Lessons

I STAND, MY GAZE SWEEPING THE ROOM, TAKING IN THE sea of faces, more than one hundred students. They look so young, Sarah's age, newly graduated from high school. Today is also her first day of classes as a college freshman. I know that, like she is, most of the students in front of me are filled with a mix of trepidation and eager anticipation.

I talk about myself in an attempt to alleviate their anxiety.

"So, yes, the accent . . . Well, it's not fake." I hear a few chuckles. "It's a mongrelized English accent." A student in the front row laughs out loud. "I was born in England, and it evolved from there."

The sound of squeaking seats is diminishing. But one student is still twirling his pencil in and around his hand, a second keeps coiling hair around her index finger, and another hasn't stopped playing with his earring.

"The short version is that I grew up in Israel." I see several of the students straighten their backs and lean forward. "Well, there were a couple of other countries and languages along the way. Like French from Switzerland, and, of course, Hebrew and Arabic from Israel . . ."

I move on to speak of dragon boating and weaving, and as I

talk, I see the fidgeting abate as these new students begin to relax in their seats, relieved that I am also a human being. They are quiet, listening, interested in me as an individual.

I pause. Is this the right time? Should I go for it?

I make eye contact with one, then another and another. They gaze back at me, their eyes intent, their focus sharp, waiting. I take a deep breath and ask, "How many of you have suffered a brain injury, including concussions?"

Silence greets me; they weren't expecting that question. A hesitant hand goes up. A rustle of movement swells as they look around the room. Another hand goes up, then two more, then four, and five. We are all turning our heads, searching. Who will be next? I wait a few moments, until the room stills.

Seats groan as the students turn back toward me and watch me expectantly, curious about my next move. More than twenty hands reach for the ceiling. Twenty percent. Twenty percent of these first-year college students have had a brain injury.

According to several studies, individuals ages fifteen to twenty-four are at the highest risk of a traumatic brain injury.

I ask some of them how they sustained their injuries.

A spiky-haired student leans back in his seat and grins as he volunteers, "A guy punched me in the face while I played water polo." Other students laugh.

I raise an eyebrow. "Does this happen to you often?" More laughter. I ask, "How long did it take you to recover?"

He shakes his head—there was no recovery time. From his description of the incident, I suspect that he did not really sustain a brain injury.

I point to a husky giant squeezed into a seat near the back. He says, "I play football. I had five concussions."

"So you haven't really recovered," I say. "Brain injury begets brain injury."

Those who sustain a brain injury are three times as likely to sustain a second injury, and those who sustain a second are eight times as likely to sustain a third.

He shrugs. "I feel fine."

I have trouble hearing another football player's tentative response. "I got a concussion a few weeks ago. I still get really bad headaches, and there's some other stuff."

I nod emphatically. "You never fully recover from a severe brain injury."

I face the entire class and square my shoulders. "I also have a brain injury. In fact, I've had three brain surgeries."

They collectively gasp and draw back in their seats.

I chuckle and add, "No worries—I don't drool or run into trees." I wait a beat as the laughter dies down. "Though I can't pass the sobriety test."

As I demonstrate that I cannot walk heel to toe without losing my balance, I tell them that in my wallet I carry a note from my neurologist stating that I'm not drunk, to show the police should they stop me while I'm behind the wheel.

Then I explain why I'm telling them about this in the first place. "I do have some residual issues, and not just the heel-to-toe thing. I get distracted easily, and I have trouble when there's too much going on around me, ADD-type stuff. In particular, I have trouble with noise, chatting. So if I ask you to be quiet, you have to be quiet; I can't teach effectively otherwise."

I was extremely anxious my first year back to teaching. Feeling vulnerable, I was reluctant to say too much about myself, let alone about the surgeries. I had trouble concentrating, especially while the students were chatting, and as a result, I did not perform as well as I should have as a teacher. I realized that I had to do something to decrease the sensory input in the classroom.

By the fall of my second year teaching, two full years after the surgeries, I felt more comfortable talking about my brain injury. As I faced the new semester, I decided to be open about the brain surgeries, using that information as a platform to convey to the students the importance of their being quiet during lectures. Nervous about my upcoming confession, I never realized that there would be other benefits to it.

The first time I spoke about my surgeries, I was shocked at the number of hands that went up in response to my question about sustained brain injuries. I got four times as many as I expected—20 percent of them had their hands raised, a rate that's been consistent through the semesters. Among the students, I saw a few mouthed "wows" and raised eyebrows; I wasn't the only one who was surprised.

I knew then that my little speech was not only about managing the noise level in the classroom but also about increasing awareness of the issues involving brain injuries. Just by asking, I immediately got a couple of messages across: brain injuries are more prevalent than one would imagine, and they happen to real people, people you might know, people like you.

My anxiety melted away. I took a couple of deep breaths and dove right in. I told them about my difficulties with reading shortly after the surgeries and about having to relearn the multiplication tables. I spoke of playing computer games for cognitive rehab and of working my way through mathematics textbooks.

I had prepared myself for the possibility that the students would greet my story with an uncomfortable silence. I had not hoped for much more than a passive response. I certainly hadn't anticipated genuine interest and was pleasantly surprised by their barrage of questions.

"Why did you need the surgeries in the first place?"

"What residual deficits do you have?"

"How long does it take to completely recover?"

On the first day of the following fall, three years postsurgery, I went through my now-usual ritual. Michael was one of the 20 percent. He sat hunched over, dark rings around his eyes, no hint of a smile on his face, even when the rest of the class was laughing. Waves of extreme anxiety and anguish rolled off him. When I asked him about his brain injury, he spoke of ongoing issues but did not elaborate.

I waited for an opportunity to speak to him. He showed up for each lecture, but he usually arrived after I was ready to start, and as soon as class was over, he was out the door.

Finally, a few weeks into the semester, he arrived earlier than usual. Busy rummaging through his backpack, he did not see me approach and was startled when he noticed me by his side. When I asked him to come see me after class, he froze and stared at me. I felt as if I had trapped a wild animal.

I smiled. "Don't worry, you're not in trouble. I just wanted to ask you about your concussion." He remained stiff. "No big deal or anything. I'm just curious."

When he came up to me after class, I asked him to accompany me to my office, thinking that it would be easier for him to talk while walking beside me, not having to make eye contact.

As we strolled side by side, I elaborated on some of my own experiences, hoping it would help him open up: my troubles with sensory overload, my issues with following directions, my depression. He nodded but volunteered nothing.

When I mentioned my difficulties initiating tasks, explaining that it was different from procrastination, he turned sharply toward me, and, for the first time since the beginning of the semester, his eyes lost their unfocused, dull look. His face became more animated. He leaned in, nodding vehemently. "I can't concentrate, and my thinking is so . . . slow."

Michael had sustained a severe concussion during football

practice, just before the beginning of the academic year. His short-term memory was affected, his attention span was really abysmal, he became overwhelmed easily, and his organizational skills had also suffered. And he was afraid and felt very much alone.

"You know that it will get better? You're not going to be stuck like this."

He looked me up and down, as if taking my measure. "The doctors told me I would get better, but . . ." He actually smiled. "But when you say it, I can believe it."

chapter thirty-one

2013 –:
See Me

PLEASE, LOOK AT ME. I'M HERE. SEE ME.

What would you do if you saw a grown woman standing in the middle of a crowd, silent, unmoving, tears streaming down her cheeks? Would you stop and try to help her?

Please, help me.

I have been that woman, and there's a real chance I will be that woman again.

We were at the Mercer County Dragon Boat Festival in New Jersey. I was there with my dragon boat team. As we always did at festivals, we chose the location for our tents carefully—we could hear the announcements clearly, yet we didn't have to raise our voices to be heard over the music.

When we left for the marshaling area to await our first race, I knew that I'd probably suffer from sensory overload—the loudspeakers were located right by the docks, colorfully attired teams were warming up vigorously, and crowds were milling around.

I knew that I should take precautions, and I had come prepared. I had brought earplugs with me, I had warned Natalie and Patty that I might have a problem, and I had explained to them how to help me. Yet I did not make the connection between theory and practice. I did not bring the earplugs with me (I left them in a safe place: my backpack), and I did not stay close to Natalie and Patty.

By the time we reached the marshaling area, it was too late. As we approached the crowds, I felt my facial muscles slacken. I knew what was coming.

Unable to initiate independent motion without guidance, I could only follow my team, my herd. I was incapable of going against the flow; I could not extricate myself from the chaos surrounding me. As we got closer to the docks, my movements became slower and stiffer. When the rest of my teammates stopped, I stopped. And became immobile.

I was trapped. The only outward sign of life in me was in my eyes. They darted around, searching for someone to help me, someone to guide me away. Everyone around me was filled with excitement, dancing with the music, laughing, yelling over the noise, but I was caught—among friends, surrounded by people who were close to me, yet alone, invisible.

Rhonda wandered over, smiling. "How are you doing, Deb? It's been a while."

I couldn't answer. I wanted help, I needed help, but I had no way of communicating my distress. I couldn't even mouth the word "help." I pleaded with my eyes. *Look at me, please.* I knew that if she really looked, she would see that something was wrong.

Rhonda and I had been good friends for several years. Though caught up in the general excitement, she was really listening. Expecting an answer and hearing none, she looked at me sharply, and she saw me.

"Deb! What's wrong? Are you okay?"

I tried to send a message from my brain to my vocal cords,

but nothing happened. My eyes teared up. All I needed to do was shake my head, even a tiny bit. I knew she'd notice. *Just shake your head. You can do it. Focus.* I focused all my energy on that one motion. *Just shake it, just a bit. Please.* But I could not.

"Deb! What's going on?"

I tried again, but my neurons wouldn't respond. I gave up. I knew that it was futile to expend any more resources on this battle. The tears spilled over. I was standing with my friend, she knew I needed help, she wanted to help me, but she didn't know how, and I had no way of enlightening her.

"Deb, talk to me. I can't help you if I don't know how. You need to tell me what I can do."

The tears flowed steadily down my cheeks. I was unable to wipe them away.

Rhonda had a niece who'd had brain stem surgery, and I'd discussed the issues of sensory overload with her quite extensively. *Please, please remember what I told you. Please make the connection.*

Rhonda's gaze seemed to be focused on a point in the distance behind me. She pursed her lips and frowned. Then I saw her brow clear and the light dawn in her eyes. "Is it the music? Is it too loud?"

I wanted to nod, but my brain wouldn't cooperate. *Can I at least blink? All I need to do is blink.* I couldn't, but it didn't matter—Rhonda nodded. She had figured it out. She knew what to do. She'd help me out of this predicament.

She scanned our surroundings and absently rubbed my back. *Don't! Oh God, don't!* I screamed silently. My nerve endings were on fire. Every motion of her hand against my back felt like she was scouring it with sandpaper. I couldn't bear it, yet I couldn't move away; I couldn't even flinch. I stood there, trapped, unable to escape the torture. The tears increased in volume, the frustration now compounded by excruciating pain. *Please stop.*

I'm begging you. I tried to catch her eye, but she wasn't looking at me. A lifetime later, she nodded and turned toward me.

Facing me, she took a step back, toward . . . where? I didn't care where she was going; all I cared about was that she had removed her hand from my back. The raw burning faded, and my brain stopped screaming. As the world swam back into focus, I was, once again, able to take in my immediate surroundings. *Where is she heading?* I tried to see beyond the hordes of people, but they were too close, crowding me, walling me off from the rest of the world. *If only I could turn my head.*

I tried to think. *She's headed away from me. She must be heading toward the outskirts of the chaos.* It was the only thing that made sense. *She wouldn't leave me stranded. Would she?* She took another step, looking back at me, beckoning with her hand. "Come on. Let's walk over there, where it isn't as loud. You'll feel better away from the noise."

I glanced at her hand, then raised my eyes to look into hers, hoping that she could read my mind. *I can't follow you. I want to, but I can't.* My brain couldn't send the signals to my body yet. Assaulted from every direction, I needed an anchor, something to ground me. *I can't on my own. Take my hand. I need to hold hands to follow you.* She didn't know; she just stood there, a few paces away from me, beckoning. *Please, just reach out and take my hand.* But she didn't.

Rhonda stepped back toward me. "Deb, I need you to tell me what I can do."

Does she think that I don't want to follow her? My tears intensified. Frustrated, she stumbled on the solution: she grabbed my hand.

"Come on."

As soon as her hand made contact with mine, I knew that it was going to be okay. I was able to follow her, slowly, haltingly, one small, shuffling step at a time. With my hand in hers, willing my feet to move, one step, then another, I was making progress. The way out of the nightmare was in sight. The tears, though decreased in volume, continued to trickle down my face. We still had a ways to go. The sensory input was still overwhelming, and I was still unable to communicate.

Every movement was laborious. I paused to rest, shifted my eyes away from my feet to Rhonda, and realized that she hadn't moved. She was standing in place, holding my hand. *Why isn't she moving? I'm following her. Why isn't she leading me? Can she not see me moving? Is my progress that slow?* She looked distracted, focusing somewhere past me. She dropped my hand. *No! Don't let go!* My feet stilled, the signals from my brain froze, no messages were getting through. The tears intensified once more.

"Deb, I'm going to talk to a couple of Pink Steel members. They're both nurses. We'll figure something out." Had she called them over? Had she beckoned?

I got the impression that Rhonda was talking to someone. I couldn't turn my head to look. Drawing on my energy reserves, I concentrated. Out of the corner of my eye, I saw that she was conversing with . . . a member of Pink Steel? She looked familiar. What were they saying? Rhonda was looking toward something or someone else. . . . Hadn't she mentioned a couple of Pink Steel members? I couldn't see who it was; she must have been standing behind me.

Rhonda turned toward me. "Deb, they're both nurses. They're here to help. They'll know what to do."

How can they know what to do? They probably don't know my story. They probably don't know about overload. But Rhonda seemed convinced that they could help. Perhaps she was right.

I stood there—what else could I do?—while Rhonda talked with them. Was she explaining to them about my issues with sensory overload? I couldn't understand their conversation, couldn't distinguish their words from the background noise, couldn't place words in sentences or sentences into meaning. I picked out the word "loud" from the noise around me. Was that Rhonda's voice?

Another lifetime later, Rhonda and the Pink Steel member within sight turned toward me. Rhonda, her brow furrowed, asked, "How about earplugs?"

I felt some of the tension in my muscles ease up. *That's it! That's exactly what I need.*

I heard a woman's voice behind me say, "I have some in my car, but it'll take too long to get them."

Rhonda's shoulders slumped. *I have some, back at the tent, in my backpack, in with my meds.* They ignored me. It took me a second to realize that I hadn't spoken out loud; then I remembered that I couldn't. The nurse I could see said, "How about toilet paper? I've got some right here."

I heard from behind me, "That'll work—we'll ball it up."

I noticed a flash of white out of the corner of my eye; then I saw a hand close around it, and, magically, a white ball of toilet paper appeared in it. It was held out toward me. *I don't think I can move my hands. I don't think I can reach out and take it.* I shrugged internally. *I'll try.* I focused on sending the signals out to my muscles and hoped for the best.

Did the fact that a resolution was in sight help? It almost felt as if hope had alleviated some of the pressure on my brain and was allowing my body to thaw. As the tension started leaving my muscles, the ban on my neurons began lifting, granting them some degree of freedom. My brain cooperated, and I managed to move in slow motion. I raised my right hand, held it out to receive the toilet paper, then moved it toward my right ear and placed the ball inside it. I couldn't apply much pressure;

my brain wouldn't allow that. Another ball appeared out of nowhere in a hand in front of me. I repeated the same process
with my left hand.

As soon as both balls were in place, the noise level diminished to a manageable degree, and within a couple of minutes, I
could feel the pressure on my brain ease up further. I experi-
mented with working my throat. I could feel the words forming
and making their way toward my tongue and lips. I spoke haltingly, softly. I managed a hint of a smile.

"I'm okay. Thanks."

And I *was* okay.

It took my mind and body a few more minutes to defrost
completely. At first, I was able to move only in slow motion and
to speak only softly, but as the minutes ticked by, the neurons
carrying messages sent by my brain sped up, and my body's re-
sponsiveness returned to normal. By the time we lined up to get
in the boat, I was fully functional, able to focus all my energy on
following the calls and paddling my heart out.

This time, I was among friends when sensory overload overcame me. Even if Rhonda hadn't come along, someone else,
another teammate, would have rescued me.

What do I do if I overload among strangers?

No one would know that I'm in trouble; no one would know
that I need help.

In most situations when I overload, I cannot communicate.
More precisely, I cannot communicate verbally. Until that incident in Mercer Park, I had assumed that my only hope was to
have with me someone who was tuned in to me, someone who
would be there to notice my plight, who would know exactly
what to do, someone like Joyce or Daniel, and now Sarah as
well. That day in Mercer Park, I learned that that is not necessarily the case. In Mercer Park, I got help from someone who

wasn't fully tuned in to me, someone who wasn't sure what to do.

Perhaps I don't need someone like Joyce with me in problematic situations. Perhaps a mere acquaintance will suffice. But I cannot limit my activities to that extent. I cannot wait for a friend to join me every time I want to go grocery shopping.

That day, I also learned that although words aren't available to me while I am in a state of extreme overload, I can still ask for help—through my tears. At Mercer Park, I communicated the same way a baby, too young for speech, communicates its needs, and Rhonda responded.

Would a complete stranger respond?

I sit here, close my eyes, and try to picture myself standing with tears streaming down my colorless, expressionless face. What would people think if they saw me like that? Would they see a crazy woman? A developmentally disabled woman? Would they see someone they'd want to avoid?

Unfortunately, in this day and age, we tend to be overly suspicious. Even people whose first instinct is to help someone in distress hesitate to become involved. We worry about overstepping our bounds, about causing trouble, about getting ourselves in trouble. Yet, even nowadays, most of us know that helping is the right thing to do.

So maybe, just maybe, if you see me standing silent, still, a vacant look on my face, tears streaming unchecked down my cheeks, you'll come up and ask, "Are you okay?" and if I'm lucky, you'll be patient and stay with me until you stumble upon a solution that leads me out of overload.

Today:
Adjusting and Readjusting

I FOLLOW THE TRAIL AS IT DIPS TOWARD HART'S RUN AND become conscious of the sound of water gurgling. The brown leaves underfoot are losing their crispness, residual moisture in the spring hollow softening them, hushing my footsteps. I pick up my pace, anticipating crossing the little wooden bridge that marks the end of the prelude to my journey and the beginning of the body of the hike.

The wood, saturated from the long winter's storms, gives almost imperceptibly when I step onto the bridge. I stand in the middle, facing upstream, watching the water buckle and bulge as it flows over and around rocks and fallen branches. A brown maple leaf disappears under the bridge. I turn to watch it reappear on the other side; I peer at the stream, willing it to emerge, but it doesn't. I wait a while longer and then give up with a twinge of disappointment.

The dull thud of my boots tramping across the bridge plays percussion for the music of the water below. Stepping down onto a bed of damp leaves makes for an abrupt transition into a new movement in the symphony surrounding me, my footsteps now barely audible.

A narrow path branches off to my right and climbs a steep slope. I hesitate for a moment, debating whether to continue along the main path or follow the less traveled track uphill. I notice a hoofprint pointing to the right. My decision made, I follow the deer tracks up the slope.

Since the surgeries, venturing out on walks, whether vigorous hikes through the woods or pleasant strolls along the river, has provided a much-needed respite from my daily struggles.

Taking the time to nourish my spirit during the academic year is imperative. But since my emotional state is closely tied to my physical issues, the greater my need for a break, the harder it is to take one. During the busiest of times at work, when fatigue shadows me wherever I go, it's almost impossible to motivate myself to actively seek this haven.

Ever since I learned of the existence of the nearby nature reserve, almost twenty years ago, I've been drawn to it, taking great pleasure in following the paths up and down the hills, hiking through various habitats, tramping across fields, following deer tracks through the hardwood forest, lingering by the pond and the stream hollow. Each season merging into the next fills me with wonder. I marvel at the changing of the leaves in the fall. I still remember the magic of standing under a canopy formed of leafless branches laden with soft clouds of snow during my first winter after the surgeries. Spring, especially May— my birth month—is my favorite time of the year. I love the thaw, when rivulets of water burble around me as I walk and new growth emerges from beneath thinning patches of snow.

I'd been meaning to come for a few weeks now, but between my continual headaches and the lousy weather, there just never seemed to be a good time.

Finally, the skies cleared and I contemplated going for a walk, but my headache, which had started as a dull pain helmeting my skull, had intensified since I'd woken, and I was afraid that any form of exertion would cause it to escalate to a crippling degree.

I tried reading, writing, and surfing the internet, but I couldn't settle into anything. The sun streaming in through the window kept beckoning. I withstood the temptation for no more than half an hour. Then I reached for my baseball cap, hoping that protecting my head from the sun and creating a band of pressure around my skull would inhibit any increase in the pain. I laced up my hiking boots, grabbed a water bottle, and set off for the nature reserve.

I follow the deer tracks uphill, the forest floor drying as I climb, the leaves growing crunchier underfoot. I crest the hill and start on my descent toward the meadow. On my way, I slow to run my hands across a moss-covered tree trunk and to stroke feather-like ferns peeking out from beneath layers of brown leaves. I meander through the shadows of a dense forest, my boots squelching in the soggy ground. The sogginess makes way for glistening mud, with deeper, sharper imprints of deer tracks. Occasionally, the muck sucks at my boots, struggling with me for ownership, then surrenders with a loud *smack*.

Every so often, I brave the thorns and the brambles alongside the trail to avoid the worst of the ooze. Whenever I come within range of the naked raspberry bushes, the hooked thorns snatch at me, snagging on my clothes and scratching my arms.

My breath catches when I come across the hoofprints of a fawn. I stop to examine them more closely, then follow them until they veer off through a gap in the bushes, broken twigs and flattened grass in their wake.

By the time I reach the meadow, the entire width of the trail is a slimy mess. Now, with every step, I have to choose which to brave: the mud or the thorns. Occasionally, a small patch of rotting leaves lends me a reprieve, allowing me to regroup before I tackle the next hindrance. An impenetrable bed of thorny bushes borders a stretch of the slippery meadow path; there is no impediment-free way. I pause, then pick my way cautiously through the oozing mud in an attempt to avoid slipping and falling. A couple of times, I do lose my footing, yet somehow, at the last minute, arms flailing, I regain my balance.

Because of the seasonality of some of my duties at work, my teaching load in the spring semester has always been greater than it is in the fall. During the fall semester, I work hard to perform well at my job. It's exhausting, but by pacing myself effectively and working around my limitations, I manage to prevent myself from slipping into the mire.

In the fall, teaching nurtures my self and gives me the inner strength I need to stay on track. When I walk into the classroom, I forget about the fatigue and overload, even on the worst of the bad brain days. The pleasure I take in my role as a teacher is well worth the price I pay for doing my job.

However, in the spring, my heavier workload drains all my resources and continues draining them as I go. I have nothing left, either physically or psychologically. Taking naps is not enough to overcome the exhaustion. The joy of interacting with my students is not sufficient to keep me going.

Every spring semester since I returned to the classroom, I have been continually exhausted, suffering from daily headaches and experiencing vertigo and precarious balance. On many days, I manage to focus through the headaches and, by moving carefully, adjusting and readjusting, to prevent loss of balance.

But there are too many days when fatigue interferes with my teaching, when I cannot focus, when my short-term memory acts up and I have trouble accessing vocabulary. There are days when an excruciating headache keeps me home, or when my balance and vertigo are so bad that I am incapable of venturing out of my office.

Every spring semester, I feel as if I am stuck in the mire, and every time the ground begins to firm under my feet, I trip over another gnarled root and fall facedown into the muck— unanticipated meetings, issues with teaching assistants, another makeup test.

A couple of years after I returned to teaching, my psychiatrist suggested that I think about going on medical disability. I was shocked at her suggestion.

Her parting words were, "Just think about it."

I thought about it. I even looked into my disability insurance, and I mentioned the idea to my neurologist during a regular checkup. I expected a noncommittal reaction, but he surprised me. "You'd certainly have our support if you decide to pursue it. With your history and symptoms . . . It's not straightforward; you'd need a lawyer. We have a couple of law offices we work with."

But I couldn't bring myself to succumb to the bloody brain. I believed that somehow I'd manage, that if I slogged through the mud, I'd eventually reach dry ground and all would be well.

Two years after my psychiatrist made her suggestion, during the semester when I taught Matrices and Linear Transformations, I was stretched far too thin. I was incapable of performing as I should have at work. My deficits, aggravated by extreme fatigue, affected my teaching. All too often, I couldn't dredge up answers to students' questions, and I had trouble working my way through the more complex math problems.

It finally sank in that the price I was paying was too dear. I couldn't keep going like this; something had to change.

In order to gain a full understanding of my options, I needed to consult with a disabilities lawyer. Although I was mo-

tivated to take action, my issues with task initiation, my pro-
longed period of recovery from the semester, and my distress
over having to take this step combined to delay my seeking a
lawyer until the fall.

I was anxious, emotional, and on the verge of overload as I
walked into the appointment at the law office. Thirty minutes
into the meeting, the emotional and sensory input got the better
of my brain. I started stuttering, had trouble focusing, lost track
of the conversation, struggled to access words, and became repetitive in my account.

After listening to my story and witnessing tangible evidence
of my deficits, the lawyer advised me to work with the university
to arrive at an agreement on accommodating my disability,
without the intervention of lawyers. He mapped out the process
for me: first undergo cognitive testing, then speak to the manager of the office of disability resources at Carnegie Mellon,
and, finally, meet with the department head.

I was still hesitant—requesting special accommodation would
require exposing the full extent of my disability to my colleagues.

For a number of years now, I'd been speaking openly of my
disability among dragon boaters, within the textile-arts community, and to students. But, like so many brain injury survivors, at
my workplace I chose to hide as much as I could about it.

I was afraid of being stigmatized, of being regarded as
lesser. I was anxious that I'd be deemed incapable of performing
my job, scared that my colleagues would question my worth as a
mathematician.

Being a mathematician is an integral part of my identity
and has been for many years. The notion of losing such an important part of who I am filled me with grief. The prospect that
the mathematical community might regard me as an outsider
was unthinkable.

I was not ready to give up my identity as a mathematician and a teacher, nor was I ready to work part-time. I knew that, under the right circumstances, I was capable of working full-time. All the evidence suggested that in order to endure, at the very least, I needed a reduction in my teaching load. Unfortunately, if my teaching load were reduced, it would quickly become common knowledge—at the beginning of each semester, every faculty member receives a copy of all the teaching assignments. By making such a request, I would be exposing my difficulties as a brain injury survivor.

I'd fought long and hard to triumph over the bloody brain and be an equal member of the faculty. And here I was, about to undo all that work, admitting defeat and, at the same time, opening myself up to resentment and pity.

But I couldn't keep going the way I had been, picking my way through the fall semester, only to land facedown in the mud every spring. I had to find a resolution. I wanted one that minimized the damage to my self-worth, did not compromise my standing among my colleagues, and allowed me to retain my identity as a mathematician.

I knew that Larry, the manager of Carnegie Mellon's office of disability resources, was a genius at coming up with simple, effective, and sometimes creative ways of providing special accommodations. He had always shown great integrity, which was important to me—I was not looking for a handout; I just wanted a fair chance at excelling at my own job.

I wanted Larry's opinion about my situation and my options. But first, following the lawyer's advice, I contacted my neuropsychologist to arrange for cognitive testing.

Because of scheduling conflicts on both our parts, I completed the testing toward the end of the fall semester and received the report a few weeks into the spring semester. By then, I was already exhibiting the usual effects of my spring workload on my neurological deficits. My usual vulnerability due to mental exhaustion was compounded by my angst over the process of resolving my situation. I was in a continual state of emotional fragility. My tears were ready to spill over at the slightest trigger. I had trouble sleeping, which aggravated the deficits further. Bad brain days became the norm.

After Larry read my neuropsychologist's report, the two of us sat down to discuss my state of affairs and options.

He kept shaking his head. "Something has to be done."

Larry explained that in the spirit of the Americans with Disabilities Act, we'd have to resolve the issue in a way that would facilitate my ability to perform my job at a level that would be acceptable to all parties involved. As I had expected, I'd probably have to take on additional duties in exchange for a reduction in teaching.

Our meeting with Tom, the department head, was scheduled for 10:30 a.m. on a Monday. I was distracted and agitated throughout the day on Sunday; when I wasn't wandering around the house without purpose, I was staring blankly at my computer screen or riffling aimlessly through books and lecture notes.

On Monday, as I waited in my office for the meeting, I pivoted in my swivel chair, every so often making an unsuccessful attempt to settle down and get some work done.

At 10:30 a.m. on the dot, I knocked on Tom's door, my hands shaking. I couldn't stop fidgeting while we waited for Larry to arrive, and throughout our meeting I kept rubbing my left thumb with my right. I had to fight to prevent my voice from quavering. I frequently clenched my teeth and swallowed to keep the moisture in my eyes from swelling into tears. "Last Friday, the headache was so bad, I had to cancel one class and find a substitute for the other. A week ago, between severe vertigo and no balance, I didn't make it to my first class. I would have needed a wheelchair to get there; a cane or a walker wouldn't have been enough."

Despite Tom's and Larry's genuine concern and their assurances that we would find a resolution, I was unable to overcome my anguish. I was overloading emotionally during the entirety of our thirty-minute meeting. I managed to hang on until the last ten minutes. By then, widening cracks in the bloody brain's veneer could no longer prevent the signs from showing. I had trouble accessing vocabulary, and I had to enunciate carefully to avoid slurring. But I stuck with it, struggling to maintain focus, to explain my situation, to suggest possible solutions to anticipated obstacles.

As we wrapped up, immense relief overpowered all my other emotions. I was hopeful for the future, hopeful that we would find a solution. But mostly I was relieved that I had managed to make it through the meeting without overloading to the point of losing my ability to move or communicate, and that my symptoms, bad as they were, hadn't made Tom or Larry uncomfortable—or made me the object of their pity.

I tried to rise from my chair, but my entire body wavered violently and I stumbled back into it. I tried again, while gripping the table in front of me, but I was incapable of standing upright. I sank back down to breathe and recover. Larry and Tom stared at me. I took a deep breath and tried again but was unsuccessful.

Both Larry and Tom offered a hand, to no avail. I sat in Tom's office, feeling frustrated and distressed. Every so often, I rose to test my balance while Tom conducted his business around me. When I finally regained some modicum of stability, instead of walking away from the meeting filled with hope, I stumbled toward my office feeling completely and utterly bereft.

I was already dispirited by my perpetual headaches; now, my misery stretched into the next week.

I knew that exercise would help disperse my mood, but I hadn't been able to exercise vigorously since my headaches had started, several weeks prior, and the weather had not been conducive to pleasant walks.

Finally, now that the sun had come out from behind the clouds and my headache was not quite crippling, I answered the call of the nature reserve.

I slowly pick my way along the muddy trail, pausing every so often to make a choice. More often than not, I opt for the mud over the thorns, venturing into them only when there is no firm purchase in the muck and my foot slips with even the most tentative of steps.

As the path climbs back out of the meadow, the mud starts drying, and I don't feel the need to step so hesitantly. The breeze picks up, awaking the trees, which creak and pop. After a while, the popping becomes more rhythmic, as if someone is knocking on a door. A couple of knocks to my right, several knocks to my left, and a few from behind—a woodpecker! It has to be a woodpecker.

I take off my hat and stand motionless, my head cocked, my eyes sweeping the bare trees, hoping for a glimpse of the bird. Unable to locate it, I move on when there is a lull in the knocking, occasionally stepping aside to avoid another patch of mud.

At a renewed series of nearby knocks, I glance upward and detect movement, something bobbing in rhythm with the knocking. I take a quiet step to the side, for a better view. And there he is, that elusive woodpecker, bobbing away, pecking at the tree trunk. I stand silently for a long moment, delighting in my discovery, and then gaze after him, following his flight, until I lose him among the trees.

Smiling, I continue toward the high ground, watching, listening. I hope for a glimpse of the bouncing patch of white as a deer bounds through the brush, or for the cry of a hawk gliding against the backdrop of the blue sky. I pause at the top of the hill to massage my temples and take in the view, the bare trees and gray branches reaching up to the sun, hiding the meadow I have left behind. I breathe the soft air, with its faint taste of moisture and light—a hint of the warmth to come. I turn to navigate the gentle slope back to my car.

Though my headache has intensified, my surroundings have dissolved the anguish that has consumed me over the last few days, replacing it with a renewed sense of self. I have replenished my long-depleted resources. Once again, I feel fully attuned to the world, to myself.

I begin the drive home at peace, content.

Without warning, three wild turkeys erupt from the woods on my left and fly across the road in front of me. My eyes zip after them as they dart into the trees and disappear.

Grinning, I turn my attention back to the road ahead.

acknowledgments

First, I'd like to thank the team at She Writes Press for transforming my manuscript into a book, especially Brooke Warner, Kamy Wicoff, Annie Tucker, Lauren Wise, Caitlyn Levin, Julie Metz, and Crystal Patriarche. Thanks also to Connie Lee, the president and founder of the Angioma Alliance, for her contribution to the book and much more. I am grateful to Judy Fort Brenneman, my writing coach and editor—an amazing teacher who pushed me to grow from a wannabe "eh" writer to a bona fide author of a book I am proud of, and became a good friend and confidante along the way.

I'd also like to acknowledge my fellow brain injury survivors worldwide, in particular the angioma community—you are one of the main reasons I started writing. I hope this book helps.

I started writing within days after I returned home from my brain surgeries, more than ten years ago. I want to express my appreciation to my neurosurgeon, the extraordinary Dr. Spetzler, and his wonderful team for giving me the chance to reclaim my life. My journey has been long, hard, and filled with wonder. I am thankful to my various support groups, including my dragon boat team, Steel City Dragons; my WARP (Weave A Real Peace) tribe; and my friends at Carnegie Mellon University. I want to mention Bill Hawthorne, Judith Patz, and Judith Diven, who put things in perspective and helped me through some of the rough patches. I am grateful to my family, Mum, Dad, Jonathan, Simon, and Rachel, who lent me strength and provided me with a shoulder whenever I needed it. And to Bill Hrusa, for his part in my healing and for caring.

I would also like to thank my loves, Daniel and Sarah, Cindy and Joyce, and, of course, Gus, for being there, always.

And finally, a nod to the Bloody Brain, my ever-present companion.

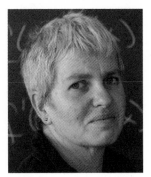

photo credit: Charlee Brodsky

Deborah (Deb) Brandon, Ph.D., has been a professor in the Mathematical Sciences Department at Carnegie Mellon University since 1991. She has participated nationally and internationally in dragon boating. She is a mother, a writer, and a respected textile artist.

Deb is also a brain injury survivor. Her journey toward reclaiming her life began with three brain surgeries. At the time, her two children were thirteen and fifteen years old.

Deb has leveraged her position as a popular and successful university professor to raise awareness of and improve understanding about brain injury. In addition to speaking openly about brain injury with more than a hundred students she teaches and advises each semester, she has been a featured speaker for and has facilitated discussions with university, medical professional, and general audiences. She is an active blogger and regularly participates in social media platforms including Facebook, where she discusses brain injury and its impact, and Twitter, where she posts observations about the sometimes absurd, sometimes bizarre, and always intriguing world of long-term brain injury survivors.

Body 2.0: Finding My Edge Through Loss and Mastectomy by Krista
Hammerbacher Haapala. $16.95, 978-1-63152-131-7. An
authentic, inspiring guide to reframing adversity that provides a
new perspective on preventative mastectomy, told through the
lens of the author's personal experience.

Beautiful Affliction: A Memoir by Lene Fogelberg. $16.95, 978-1-
63152-985-6. The true story of a young woman's struggle to
raise a family while her body slowly deteriorates as the result of
an undetected fatal heart disease.

A Leg to Stand On: An Amputee's Walk into Motherhood by Colleen
Haggerty. $16.95, 978-1-63152-923-8. Haggerty's candid story
of how she overcame the pain of losing a leg at seventeen—and
of terminating two pregnancies as a young woman—and went
on to become a mother, despite her fears.

Her Beautiful Brain: A Memoir by Ann Hedreen. $16.95, 978-1-
938314-92-6. The heartbreaking story of a daughter's experiences as her beautiful, brainy mother begins to lose her mind to
an unforgiving disease: Alzheimer's.

Green Nails and Other Acts of Rebellion: Life After Loss by Elaine So-
loway. $16.95, 978-1-63152-919-1. An honest, often humorous
account of the joys and pains of caregiving for a loved one with
a debilitating illness.

Naked Mountain: A Memoir by Marcia Mabee. $16.95, 978-1-
63152-097-6. A compelling memoir of one woman's journey of
natural world discovery, tragedy, and the enduring bonds of
marriage, set against the backdrop of a stunning mountaintop in
rural Virginia.